ns and Sexes in the TCGA Data**

Colorectal & Hernia Laparoscopic Surgery

Emeka Ray-Offor • Raul J. Rosenthal
Editors

Colorectal & Hernia Laparoscopic Surgery

Principles & Practice

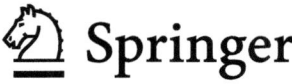 Springer

Editors
Emeka Ray-Offor
College of Health Sciences
University of Port Harcourt Choba
Rivers State, Nigeria

Raul J. Rosenthal
Department of General Surgery
Cleveland Clinic Florida
Weston, FL, USA

ISBN 978-3-031-63489-5   ISBN 978-3-031-63490-1 (eBook)
https://doi.org/10.1007/978-3-031-63490-1

© The Editor(s) (if applicable) and The Author(s), under exclusive license to Springer Nature Switzerland AG 2024

This work is subject to copyright. All rights are solely and exclusively licensed by the Publisher, whether the whole or part of the material is concerned, specifically the rights of translation, reprinting, reuse of illustrations, recitation, broadcasting, reproduction on microfilms or in any other physical way, and transmission or information storage and retrieval, electronic adaptation, computer software, or by similar or dissimilar methodology now known or hereafter developed.

The use of general descriptive names, registered names, trademarks, service marks, etc. in this publication does not imply, even in the absence of a specific statement, that such names are exempt from the relevant protective laws and regulations and therefore free for general use.

The publisher, the authors and the editors are safe to assume that the advice and information in this book are believed to be true and accurate at the date of publication. Neither the publisher nor the authors or the editors give a warranty, expressed or implied, with respect to the material contained herein or for any errors or omissions that may have been made. The publisher remains neutral with regard to jurisdictional claims in published maps and institutional affiliations.

This Springer imprint is published by the registered company Springer Nature Switzerland AG
The registered company address is: Gewerbestrasse 11, 6330 Cham, Switzerland

If disposing of this product, please recycle the paper.

Foreword

It is with immense pleasure that I author this foreword for Drs. Ray-Offor and Rosenthal. The prerequisites for success for any textbook are the depth and breadth of content, the expertise of the authors, and the relevance to the reader. This textbook by Drs. Ray-Offor and Rosenthal not only fulfill but exceed expectations in each of these areas. They have selected exceptionally timely topics which have been authoritatively written by internationally acclaimed experts. Furthermore, they have ensured that each selected topic is of tremendous current relevance and that the contents within each contribution are readily translatable into every reader's clinical practice. Moreover, to further facilitate the adoption of the outstanding principles included in these comprehensive in-depth chapters they have ensured illustrations and references to ensure the success of every reader in this goal. I am delighted to see this team working together to bring this important volume of work to the public domain. Drs. Ray-Offor and Rosenthal have combined talents from throughout the world to bring the reader 15 expertly written, comprehensibly referenced, and well-illustrated chapters outlining the gamut of laparoscopic procedures performed for the colon and rectum as well as for hernias. The first section of their book includes laparoscopy for the small and large bowel, the second and largest section focuses on the rectum, while the third section on the pelvic floor transitions towards hernias with the chapter on laparoscopic ventral rectopexy. Ultimately, the fourth section includes four superlative chapters on laparoscopic hernia repair. Recognizing that there are many textbooks available to surgeons, I enthusiastically commend to you this textbook—*Colorectal/Hernia Laparoscopic Surgery: Principles and Practice*. The internationally esteemed authors selected by Drs. Rosenthal and Ray-Offor have shared with us their unique important insights into the management of these conditions. Their technique of writing and illustration as well as the references provided are a resource for practicing general, laparoscopic, hernia, and colorectal surgeons and trainees.

I congratulate my dear friends, Drs. Ray-Offor and Rosenthal as well as all of the chapter authors on this phenomenal work. I thank them for allowing me to author this foreword.

Weston, FL, USA   Steven D. Wexner
Cleveland, OH, USA
Boca Raton, USA
Miami, FL, USA
Tampa, FL, USA
London, UK

Preface

A notable advancement in abdominal surgery has been the incorporation of optics, video technology, and unique instruments which are applied through miniature incisions on the abdominal skin to perform diagnostic and therapeutic operations. This technique of minimally invasive surgery (laparoscopy) as performed in a closed cavity with precision is associated with reduced post-operative pain, early recovery, shorter hospital stays, and time to resume work duties.

The application, interest, and enthusiasm for laparoscopic surgery have remarkably increased, across surgical specialties. In colorectal surgery, there are technically simple surgeries (e.g. colostomy and ileostomy) and complex surgeries including colectomies, and rectal and pelvic floor surgeries. Additionally, there are transanal endoscopic approaches for disease management. Hernias are complications of abdominal surgeries including stoma creation and they often require surgical repair. These surgeries can be performed through a laparoscopic approach with all the attendant benefits of minimally invasive surgery.

Competence in laparoscopic colorectal and hernia surgeries like every new technology requires training. This book contains a concise and in-depth discussion of the key aspects of performing laparoscopic colorectal and hernia surgeries—introduction, relevant anatomy, indications, and contraindications, preoperative preparation, technique of surgery, post-operative care with special notes on the practice. This is designed as an up-to-date guidebook for surgeons with privileges to perform these surgeries and an aid to proctored training for trainees in colorectal, hernia, and general surgeons. It is our sincere hope that this book meets the stated expectations.

Port Harcourt, Nigeria Emeka Ray-Offor
Weston, FL, USA Raul J. Rosenthal

Contents

Part I Small Bowel/Colon

1. **Laparoscopic Ileostomy** 3
   Emeka Ray-Offor, Peter Rogers, and Zoe Garoufalia

2. **Laparoscopic Colostomy** 15
   Emeka Ray-Offor, Elisa Cassinotti, Ludovica Baldari,
   and Luigi Boni

3. **Laparoscopic Colectomy** 23
   Olusegun Komolafe

4. **Robot-Assisted Laparoscopic Colorectal Surgery** 39
   Emeka Ray-Offor and Olusegun Komolafe

Part II Rectum

5. **Laparoscopic Anterior Resection** 51
   Emeka Ray-Offor, Sameh Hany Emile, and Nir Horesh

6. **Laparoscopic Abdominoperineal Resection** 65
   Emeka Ray-Offor, Nir Horesh, and Sameh Hany Emile

7. **Laparoscopic Restorative Proctectomy with Ileal Pouch-Anal
   Anastomosis**... 75
   Olusegun Komolafe

8. **Transanal Endoscopic Microsurgery** 85
   Emeka Ray-Offor

9. **Transanal Minimally Invasive Surgery TAMIS** 93
   Matthew Albert and Paul M. Kaminsky

10. **Transanal Total Mesorectal Excision** 107
    Emeka Ray-Offor and Victor Strassmann

Part III Pelvic Floor

11 **Laparoscopic Ventral Rectopexy** 119
    Mukhtar Ahmad

Part IV Hernia

12 **Laparoscopic Ventral Hernia Repair** 129
    Emeka Ray-Offor and Raul J. Rosenthal

13 **Laparoscopic Parastomal Hernia Repair** 137
    Emeka Ray-Offor, Emanuele Lo Menzo, Samuel Szomstein,
    and Raul J. Rosenthal

14 **Transabdominal Preperitoneal Hernia Repair (TAPP)** 145
    Usman Mohammed Bello

15 **Totally Extraperitoneal Hernia Repair** 157
    Yin Min Benjamin Tan, Samuel Szomstein, Emanuele Lo Menzo,
    and Raul J. Rosenthal

Index 167

Editors and Contributors

About the Editors

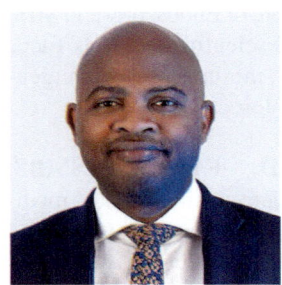

Emeka Ray-Offor, MBBS(Nig) FWACS FMAS DMAS FACS An astute surgeon skilled in Endoscopy, Minimally Invasive Surgery, and Colorectal and Hernia surgeries with a Bachelor of Medicine, Bachelor of Surgery degree-MBBS, from the University of Nigeria, Nsukka, and postgraduate surgery training acquired in India, Europe, and the USA. He recently completed a 1-year Research Fellowship in the Colorectal Surgery department of Ellen Leifer Shulman and Steven Shulman Digestive Disease Center, Cleveland Clinic Florida, USA. He has held a faculty position in the College of Health Science, University of Port Harcourt, Choba, Rivers State, Nigeria, since 2011 and is currently a Professor of General and Minimal Access Surgery. In addition, he is the Director of Minimal Access Surgery Program at the University of Port Harcourt Teaching Hospital, Port Harcourt, Rivers State, Nigeria, an Honorary Consultant General and Minimally Invasive Surgeon in the Colorectal/Minimal Access Surgery Unit, Department of Surgery and Lead, Gastrointestinal Cancer Multi-Disciplinary Team of the hospital.

Professor Ray-Offor is a surgeon educator and has organized multiple workshops for training in Endoscopy/Minimal Access Surgery. He is a seasoned author with over 80 abstracts and peer-reviewed journal publications, in addition to being the editor of two books on Endoscopy and Laparoscopic surgery, respectively. He is a reviewer of multiple scientific journals and a member of the Editorial Board/Co-editor of the Nigerian *Journal of Gastroenterology and Hepatology* with membership in several professional societies in Africa, Europe, Asia, and North America. These include the West African College of Surgeons (WACS), the Society for Gastroenterology and Hepatology (SOGHIN), the Nigerian Society for Colorectal Disorders (NSCD), the European Association for Endoscopic Surgeons (EAES), the World Association of Laparoscopic Surgeons (WALS), the American College of Surgeons (ACS), the Society of American Gastrointestinal Endoscopic Surgeons (SAGES), and the American Society of Colon and Rectal Surgeons (ASCRS).

He is the founder of Oak Endoscopy Centre & Radiodiagnostics, Port Harcourt, Nigeria—a non-profit organization for the advancement of Endoscopy and MIS.

His main professional and scientific interests focus on gastrointestinal endoscopy, minimally invasive general/colorectal surgery, and colorectal cancer.

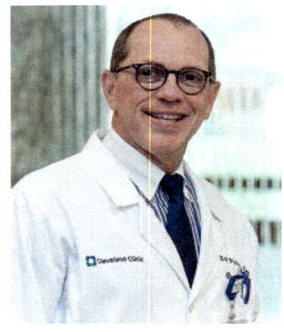

Raul J. Rosenthal, MD, FACS, FASMBS, MAMSE is an industry leader, prolific author, medical researcher, and attending surgeon at Cleveland Clinic Florida, where he has conducted well over 10,000 general surgery and bariatric procedures and trained more than 50 fellows in advanced gastrointestinal, minimally invasive, and bariatric surgery. In 2018, Dr Rosenthal received the LEAD Award from the American Society of Metabolic & Bariatric Surgery (ASMBS) Foundation in recognition of lifetime contributions to the field of bariatric surgery. Also in 2018, his breakthrough research into the use of indocyanine green fluorescence imaging in laparoscopic cholecystectomy was featured during the American College of Surgeons (ACS) annual Clinical Congress. Based on the results of Dr Rosenthal's multinational, multi-year trial, the use of fluorescence imaging is becoming established as the gold standard of care for minimally invasive gall bladder removal and other abdominal procedures worldwide.

Dr Rosenthal completed his medical school and surgical residency in Rosario, Argentina. In 1982, after emigrating to Frankfurt, Germany, and repeating a general surgery residency, he became an attending surgeon at the Northwest Hospital. In 1993, Dr Rosenthal emigrated to the USA, where 3 years of minimally invasive surgery fellowship at Cedars-Sinai Medical Center in LA were followed by a third general surgery residency at Mount Sinai Medical Center in New York City. After arriving at Cleveland Clinic Florida, Dr Rosenthal became Chief of Minimally Invasive and Bariatric Surgery and Director of the Fellowship program. He has subsequently served as Chief of the Medical Staff, Chairman of the Department of General Surgery, Director of the General Surgery Residency Program, and Chairman of the Medical Executive Committee. Among his professional leadership roles, Dr Rosenthal served as president of the Society of American Gastrointestinal and Endoscopic Surgeons (SAGES) and the SAGES Foundation; and as a past president of the executive committee of the ASMBS and the ASMBS Foundation. Dr Rosenthal is founding Clinical Editor of Bariatric Times and Associate Editor of SOARD and Obesity Surgery. He serves as the Editorial Board member of Annals of Surgery, Selected Readings in General Surgery Langenbeck's Archives of Surgery, and Surgical Endoscopy. He is a founding member and a past President of the Fellowship Council and also served as President of the South Florida Chapter of the ACS and Governor of the ACS.

A polyglot, Dr Rosenthal is fluent in English, Spanish, and German. He has been granted honorary membership by professional organizations around the world, including the Federation of Latin American Surgeons, and the Argentinian, Indian, Peruvian, German, and Israeli Societies of Surgery. Dr Rosenthal is the author or co-author of over 300 abstracts and peer-reviewed publications, more than 30 book chapters, and over 100 educational videos. He has contributed over 80 book chapters and is the Co-Editor of several books including the ASMBS *Textbook of Bariatric Surgery*, *Globesity*, *Netter's Gastroenterology*, *The Pathophysiology of Pneumoperitoneum*, *Fluorescence Imaging for Surgeons*, *Operative Strategies in Laparoscopic Surgery*, *Weight Loss Surgery and Mental Conditioning to Perform Common Operations in General Surgery Training: A Systematic Approach to Expediting Skill Acquisition and Maintaining Dexterity in Performance*.

Contributors

Mukhtar Ahmad, MMedSci FRCS Consultant General and Colorectal Surgeon, University Hospitals, Dorset, UK

Matthew Albert, MD FACS FASCRS Professor of Surgery, Advent Health Medical Group, Center for Colon and Rectal Surgery, Orlando, FL, USA

Ludovica Baldari, MD Consultant Surgeon, General and Minimally Invasive Surgery, Fondazione IRCCS—Ca' Granda—Ospedale Maggiore, Policlinico di Milano, Milan, Italy

Usman Mohammed Bello, MBBS FWACS Consultant Surgeon, Aminu Kano Teaching Hospital, Kano, Kano State, Nigeria

Senior Lecturer, Bayero University, Kano, Kano State, Nigeria

Luigi Boni, MD FRCS FACS Professor of Surgery, University of Milan, Milan, Italy

Chief of General and Minimally Invasive Surgery, Fondazione IRCCS—Ca' Granda—Ospedale Maggiore, Policlinico di Milano, Milan, Italy

Elisa Cassinotti, MD PhD Clinical Resercher, University of Milan, Milan, Italy

Consultant Surgeon, General and Minimally Invasive Surgery, Fondazione IRCCS—Ca' Granda—Ospedale Maggiore, Policlinico di Milano, Milan, Italy

Sameh Hany Emile, MBBCh MSc MD/PhD FACS Project Scientist, Colorectal Surgery Department, Ellen Leifer Shulman and Steven Shulman Digestive Disease Institute, Cleveland Clinic Florida, Weston, FL, USA

Associate Professor and Consultant of General and Colorectal Surgery, Department of General Surgery, Faculty of Medicine, Mansoura University, Mansoura, Egypt

Clinical Affiliate Associate Professor of Surgery, Schmidt College of Medicine, Florida Atlantic University, Boca Raton, FL, USA

Zoe Garoufalia, MD Minimally Invasive Colon and Rectal Surgery Fellow, Colorectal Surgery Department, Ellen Leifer Shulman and Steven Shulman Digestive Disease Institute, Cleveland Clinic, Weston, FL, USA

Nir Horesh, MD Advanced Minimally Invasive Colorectal Surgery Fellow, Colorectal Surgery Department, Ellen Leifer Shulman and Steven Shulman Digestive Disease Institute, Cleveland Clinic Florida, Weston, FL, USA

Assistant Professor, Faculty of Medicine, Tel Aviv University, Tel Aviv, Israel

Paul M. Kaminsky, MD PhD Colorectal Surgeon, Advent Health Medical Group, Center for Colon and Rectal Surgery, Orlando, FL, USA

Olusegun Komolafe, FRCS Consultant General and Colorectal Surgeon, University Hospital Wishaw, Wishaw, Scotland

Honorary Clinical Senior Lecturer, University of Glasgow, Glasgow, Scotland

Editors and Contributors

David Maron, MD FACS FASCRS Vice Chair/Attending Colorectal Surgeon, Department of Colorectal Surgery, Attending Colorectal Surgeon, Ellen Leifer Shulman and Steven Shulman Digestive Disease Center, Cleveland Clinic Florida, Weston, FL, USA

Emanuele Lo Menzo, MD PhD FACS FASMBS Vice Chairman/Associate Program Director, General Surgery Residency Program, Department of General Surgery, Program Cleveland Clinic Florida, The Bariatric and Metabolic Institute, Ellen Leifer Shulman and Steven Shulman Digestive Disease Center, Weston, FL, USA

Clinical Affiliate Professor, Charles E. Schmidt College of Medicine, Florida Atlantic University, Boca Raton, FL, USA

Clinical Associate Professor, Herbert Wertheim College of Medicine, Florida International University, Miami, FL, USA

Austin Obichere, MD FRCS Director Bowel Cancer Screening Program/Consultant Colorectal Surgeon, University College London Hospital, London, UK

Emeka Ray-Offor, MBBS(Nig) FWACS FMAS DMAS FACS Professor of Surgery, College of Health Sciences, University of Port Harcourt, Choba, Rivers State, Nigeria

Honorary Consultant General and Minimally Invasive Surgeon, Colorectal/Minimal Access Surgery Unit, Department of Surgery, University of Port Harcourt Teaching Hospital, Port Harcourt, Rivers State, Nigeria

Founder/ Lead Endoscopic Surgeon, Digestive Disease Unit, Oak Endoscopy Centre, Port Harcourt, Rivers State, Nigeria

Peter Rogers, MD Research Fellow, Colorectal Surgery Department, Ellen Leifer Shulman and Steven Shulman Digestive Disease Institute, Cleveland Clinic, Weston, FL, USA

Raul J. Rosenthal, MD FACS FASMBS MAMSE Regional Vice Chief, Ellen Leifer Shulman and Steven Shulman Digestive Disease Institute, Cleveland Clinic Florida, Weston, FL, USA

Regional Chair and Director General Surgery Residency Program, Division of General Surgery, Cleveland Clinic Florida, Weston, FL, USA

Director, The Bariatric and Metabolic Institute, Ellen Leifer Shulman and Steven Shulman Digestive Disease Center, Cleveland Clinic Florida, Weston, FL, USA

Clinical Professor of Surgery, Cleveland Clinic Lerner College of Medicine at Case Western Reserve University, Cleveland, OH, USA

Clinical Affiliate Professor, Charles E. Schmidt College of Medicine, Florida Atlantic University, Boca Raton, FL, USA

Clinical Professor, Herbert Wertheim College of Medicine, Florida International University, Miami, FL, USA

Dana Sands, MD FASCRS Attending Colorectal Surgeon, Department of Colorectal Surgery, Ellen Leifer Shulman and Steven Shulman Digestive Disease Center, Cleveland Clinic Florida, Weston, FL, USA

Victor Strassmann, MD PhD Clinical Research Associate, Department of Colorectal Surgery, Ellen Leifer Shulman and Steven Shulman Digestive Disease Institute, Cleveland Clinic Florida, Weston, FL, USA

Patricia Sylla, MD FACS FASCRS Chief of Colon and Rectal Surgery and President, Society of American gastrointestinal and Endoscopic Surgeons (SAGES), Mount Sinai Hospital, New York, NY, USA

Samuel Szomstein, MD FACS FASMBS Director Minimally Invasive Surgery/Bariatric Fellowship, Department of General Surgery, The Bariatric and Metabolic Institute, Ellen Leifer Shulman and Steven Shulman Digestive Disease Center, Cleveland Clinic Florida, Weston, FL, USA

Clinical Associate Professor, Herbert Wertheim College of Medicine, Florida International University, Miami, FL, USA

Yin Min Benjamin Tan, MD Advanced General/Minimal Invasive Surgeon, General, Minimally Invasive and Bariatric Surgery, Cleveland Clinic Florida, Weston, FL, USA

Steven D. Wexner, MD, PhD (Hon), FACS, FRCS (Eng), FRCS(Ed), FRCSI (Hon), Hon FRCS (Glasg), Hon FRCS (Eng), MAMSE Emeritus Chair, Department of Colorectal Surgery, Ellen Leifer Shulman, and Steven Shulman Digestive Disease Center, Cleveland Clinic Florida, Weston, FL, USA

Clinical Professor, Cleveland Clinic Lerner College of Medicine at Case Western Reserve University, Cleveland, OH, USA

Clinical Affiliate Professor, Charles E. Schmidt College of Medicine, Florida Atlantic University, Boca Raton, FL, USA

Clinical Professor, Herbert Wertheim College of Medicine, Florida International University, Miami, FL, USA

Affiliate Professor, Department of Surgery, University of South Florida Morsani College of Medicine, Tampa, FL, USA

Honorary Professor, Division of Surgery, and Interventional Science, Department of Targeted Intervention, University College London, London, UK

Visiting Professor, Department of Surgery and Cancer, Imperial College London, London, UK

Part I
Small Bowel/Colon

Chapter 1
Laparoscopic Ileostomy

Emeka Ray-Offor, Peter Rogers, and Zoe Garoufalia

Introduction

Ileostomy, the surgical creation of an artificial opening in the abdominal wall to redirect the ileal lumen, is a common operation in the colorectal surgeon's workload. In the United States alone, about 40,000 new ileostomies are performed annually and an average of 215,000 individuals have an ileostomy at any given time [1]. Ileostomy creation has evolved in technique and indications since the pioneering work of German surgeon, Baum, in 1879 to divert an obstructing carcinoma of the right colon [2]. In current practice, a stoma is created in an acute or elective setting to protect a distal anastomosis, relieve a distal obstruction, or divert stool from pelvic or perianal/perineal sepsis [3]. Careful identification of patient and technical factors linked with the risk of anastomotic leakage are critical, as approximately half of diverting stomas are not eventually reversed and will become permanent stomas [4].

The choice between a loop ileostomy and transverse colostomy for fecal diversion is highly debatable. Evidence from the literature favors the use of loop ileostomy based on reports of lower risk of prolapse and infectious complications, in addition to an improved patient experience [4, 5]. Conversely, a loop transverse colostomy could be a preferred choice for older patients to avoid electrolyte

E. Ray-Offor (✉)
Colorectal/Minimal Access Surgery Unit, Department of Surgery, University of Port Harcourt Teaching Hospital, Port Harcourt, Rivers State, Nigeria

College of Health Sciences, University of Port Harcourt, Choba, Rivers State, Nigeria
e-mail: emeka.ray-offor@uniport.edu.ng

P. Rogers · Z. Garoufalia
Colorectal Surgery Department, Ellen Leifer Shulman and Steven Shulman Digestive Disease Institute, Cleveland Clinic Florida, Weston, FL, USA

imbalance and renal insufficiency [6]. The use of the laparoscopic approach for stoma creation is technically feasible and can be performed with low morbidity [7]. Though a low-risk surgical procedure from a technical standpoint, it carries substantial postoperative morbidity that can greatly hamper patients' quality of life and recovery. Complications can be minimized by paying careful attention to detail when surgically creating an ileostomy and follow-up care.

The decision to proceed with a stoma should be highly individualized, one that carefully weighs the negative impact on role and function against the benefits of minimizing leak complications [8]. Notably, a dedicated intestinal stoma education program and the team highly improve patients' quality of life, proficiency in patient management of stoma, reduced length of stay, reduced hospital costs, and increased psychosocial adjustment [9].

Relevant Anatomy

The small intestine starts from the duodenum, is retroperitoneally located, and ends at the ileocaecal valve. It has an approximate length of 7 meters. The other segments (jejunum and ileum) are suspended intraperitoneally by a mesentery containing their blood vessels, lymphatics, and nerves. It is important to note that the more distal the stoma site the less likelihood of impaired nutrient absorption, hence the jejunum is rarely used for stoma creation.

In performing an ileostomy, a well-vascularized segment of the ileum, without tension, is exteriorized through a trephine incision on a marked skin site of the anterior abdominal wall. Typically, the right lower abdomen is selected; however, in obese patients, visibility is often best by situating the stoma above the umbilicus. An ileostomy can be created in an end or loop configuration. An end ileostomy has a completely divided ileal segment with the entire circumference of the lumen attached 'end on' to the skin of the anterior abdominal wall. Usually, this will serve as a permanent stoma. Loop ileostomy creation exteriorizes a 'knuckle' of ileum which is opened to form 2 lumens with an intact posterior wall. The proximal limb effluent is stool, while the distal limb usually acts as a mucous fistula, draining out the secretions produced within the mucosal lining from the lumen to the caecum. Other configurations are double barrel and continent ileostomies. It is important to spout the stump to get the effluent away from contact with the skin.

For ileostomy site selection, it is recommended that an end ileostomy traverses the rectus abdominus muscle to reduce the risk of parastomal hernia formation and prolapse. When sited superior to the arcuate line the bowel segment traverses outwardly the parietal peritoneum, transversalis fascia, posterior rectus sheath, and muscle, shy of the inferior epigastric vessel then the anterior rectus sheath, passing through the trephine skin incision via the subcutaneous layers (Campers and

Scarpa's fascia). A more lateral site can be chosen like the anterior abdominal wall muscles at the edge of the rectus sheath. The structures traversed outwardly are the parietal peritoneum, transversalis fascia, transversus abdominus, internal oblique, external oblique fascia, the subcutaneous layers, and skin.

A competent ileocaecal valve prevents decompression of the colon during a large bowel obstruction, with the risk of perforation from a closed-loop obstruction.

Indications

Generally, an ileostomy is used to divert the fecal stream in various settings which include:

1. Protection of low rectal anastomosis from septic complications

    A temporary diverting loop ileostomy is usually created to obviate the impact of pelvic sepsis complicating an anastomotic leakage. The identified high-risk patients that reap the greatest benefit from fecal diversion include those with advanced age, male sex, obesity, cardiovascular comorbidities, corticosteroid use, malnutrition, clinical obstruction, preoperative chemoradiotherapy, transfusion, contamination of the operative field, technical failures, and anastomosis 5 cm from the anal verge [10–12].

2. To divert stool from pelvic or perianal/perineal sepsis

    An ileostomy may be used to divert the fecal stream in the management of complex perianal sepsis and fistulas in Crohn's disease, diverticulitis, and for healing of perineal pressure ulcers [13].

3. To divert stool in the management of fecal incontinence

    In the management of fecal incontinence, before anal sphincter reconstructive surgery, sometimes a stoma is required for diversion.

4. To permanently divert the fecal stream

    A permanent ileostomy is used in settings where a restorative procedure is not possible. This includes operations like total proctocolectomy for a patient with familial adenomatous polyposis, ulcerative colitis, or Crohn's disease. Also, following an ileoanal pouch excision.

Contraindications

There are no absolute contraindications for the creation of ileostomies in colorectal surgery. Relative contraindications are when this creation is not technically feasible, like a short mesentery under tension or failed mobilization in the setting of carcinomatosis.

Preoperative Preparation

A full clinical evaluation is made, the patient is counseled on the reasons for their stoma, and informed consent is obtained. Ideally, the stoma site is preoperatively marked by a stoma therapist in all cases. Colorectal surgeons should be familiar with the preoperative assessment for ileostomy because, in the emergent setting, stoma therapists may not be available to mark the stoma site. Consideration is made to center the marking at a readily visible site in multiple positions with a 2-inch flat healthy surrounding surface away from skin creases, bony prominences, scars, and incision wounds. The marking is done following an inspection in several positions including prone, sitting, standing, and leaning forward noting abdominal skin folds. These folds can affect the proper fitting of appliances leading to leakage and skin complications. There are better functional outcomes, less morbidity, and improved quality of life associated with a well-placed ileostomy.

Two sets of equipment are required for the laparoscopic aspect of surgery. The laparoscope and optical system, three trocars (10–12 mm), laparoscopic scissors, two Babcock forceps, dissecting forceps, and an energy device. An appropriate open surgery set is needed for the trephination.

Mechanical bowel preparation in some cases may be administered, but perioperative administration of a third-generation cephalosporin/metronidazole is mandatory.

Technique

Following induction of adequate general anesthesia with endotracheal intubation, the patient is carefully positioned in the modified lithotomy position, depending on the exact operation. Great care is taken to carefully pad and protect all areas of potential body injury. The abdomen, pelvis, and perineum are prepped and draped in a usual sterile manner.

An infraumbilical vertical incision is made through which a 10 mm Hasson cannula is carefully placed. Carbon dioxide pneumoperitoneum of 12–15 mmHg is achieved. A second 10 mm cannula is carefully placed under direct vision through a horizontal stab wound in the previously identified right lower abdominal ileostomy site. An initial diagnostic laparoscopy is performed. A third port is placed in a contralateral position relative to the stoma site and is used to mobilize the bowel and possibly divide adhesions.

Loop Ileostomy

With the 10 mm diameter Babcock grasping forceps that is inserted into the port at the marked site, a loop of distal ileum about 12–15 cm from the ileocecal valve which would easily reach above skin level in a tension-free manner is grasped and carefully maintained in its appropriate anatomic orientation.

Capnoperitoneum is released, then the aperture in the abdominal wall is created by excising a 2 cm disk of skin and incising the underlying fat and anterior rectus sheath in a cephalad to caudad direction. The rectus fibers are spread along their axis and the posterior sheath and peritoneum are incised in cephalad to caudad direction. The loop of the ileum grasped by the Babcock forceps is gently delivered through the stoma site such that 5 cm rests above the skin in a tension-free manner (Fig. 1.1).

Some surgeons place a rod in a mesenteric window in the exteriorized bowel loop and suture it in place with 2-0 silk. However, evidence from an RCT comparing ileostomies fashioned with a rigid bridge versus no bridge did not demonstrate any significant difference in early retraction rates (Fig. 1.2) [14].

Capnoperitoneum is then reestablished and an inspection with the laparoscope is made to ensure that the ileostomy has not twisted and that the correct orientation of proximal and distal limbs is maintained. The abdomen is desufflated as the umbilical port site and third port are closed. The ileostomy is then matured by incising with electrocautery, flush on the efferent limb opening about three-quarters of the ileal circumference. Using 3-0 chromic, six to eight everting maturation sutures are applied taking full-thickness bites of the cut edge, seromuscular bites at skin level, and intracuticular bites of skin.

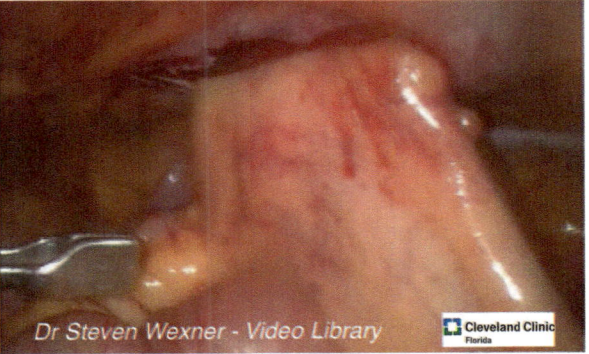

Fig. 1.1 Laparoscopic view of externalized bowel loop

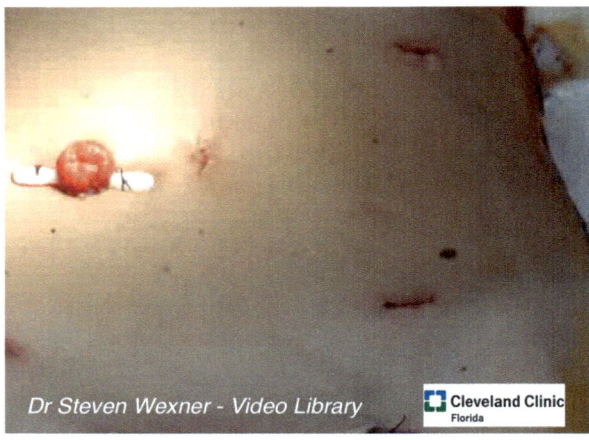

Fig. 1.2 Loop ileostomy with a rigid bride

End Ileostomy

For this configuration, an end ileostomy, the trephine is similarly created. The stapled end of the ileum is brought out through the created abdominal wall defect with usual laparoscopic checks for rotation of the end limb. The stapled end is excised, and everting maturation sutures are applied taking full-thickness bites of the cut edge, seromuscular bites at skin level, and intracuticular bites of skin at 4 poles and securing the interrupted sutures using square knots. When the mesentery is short, or the pannus of the anterior abdominal wall forestalls a non-tension stoma, construction of a loop can be created with the stapled bowel segment-

An appliance is then placed over the healthy, pink, well everted stoma. The patient is then moved from the theatre to the recovery room.

Postoperative Care

Typically, ileostomies become functional after 24 hours from construction. Regular inspection of stoma mucosa is needed in the immediate post-operative period hence it is preferable to use transparent stoma appliances. Close monitoring of body weight, fluid balance, serum biochemistry, and electrolytes are mandatory. Patients need adequate education, training, and psychosocial support to successfully adapt to stoma-related self-care [15]. Despite advances in surgery, complications of stomas remain high with risk factors that can be patient, disease, or procedure-centered. It is important to note that most of the complications are preventable by paying attention to site selection as improper siting leads to difficulties in self-care and interferes with the ability to maintain a secure stoma appliance.

Stoma complications are grouped as early or late. The former occurs within 30 days of stoma creation and includes vascular compromise, nonfunctioning of the stoma, mucocutaneous separation, retraction, high-output fistula, and skin excoriation [16]. A detailed discussion on the management of stomas is beyond the scope of this book, however, some highlights are now shared.

Vascular Compromise

An interruption of segmental arterial supply to the exteriorized segment of the bowel may occur. This can be due to tightness of the abdominal wall trephine, tension on the bowel mesentery, excessive dissection of the peristomal mesentery, or ligation of the primary blood vessel, all of which can lead to ischemia. Ischemia, which can progress to necrosis, usually develops within 24 hours of the procedure. This can be detected with a simple inspection of the stoma, demonstrating mucosa as a bluish discoloration at the mucocutaneous junction. It is pertinent to ascertain if necrosis is above or below the abdominal fascia using endoscopy through the stoma site. The former can be expectantly managed, while necrosis more than 1–2 cm, or below the fascia requires surgical revision.

Mucocutaneous Separation

Patient-related risk factors for mucocutaneous separation include infection, diabetes mellitus, corticosteroids, malnutrition, excessive tension at the stoma, and stoma necrosis [17]. Mucocutaneous separation is managed expectantly by local wound care. This involves irrigation of the separated area with saline and applying skin barrier powder. The latter can absorb exudates and fill the defect before applying the pouching system. In the case of deep separation, this can be filled with alginate or gelling fiber, then hydrocolloid dressing is applied.

Non-functioning Stoma

The procedure-centered factors that may result in the non-functioning of a stoma include an inadvertently closed stoma or maturation of a stoma with the wrong end up. These can mimic a prolonged postoperative ileus or a distal bowel obstruction. Additionally, an improper alignment of limbs may result in bowel obstruction. Radiological evaluation comprising a gentle water-soluble contrast enema via the stoma is useful to evaluate for technical error and a confirmation of this mandates surgical correction.

High Output Stoma

An ileostomy usually produces around 500–1000 mls/day, which is initially bilious and watery. Typically, the effluent thickens and becomes soft in consistency as the diet progresses; however, this may be altered by food and fluid intake, medications, active Crohn's disease, adhesions, and radiation therapy [2]. When the effluent exceeds 1500 mls, it is considered excessive and predisposes such patients to dehydration, electrolyte imbalance (hypokalaemia/ hypomagnesemia), and acute kidney injury. Dehydration from high output stoma is a major cause of readmission after stoma creation.

Skin Excoriation

The leakage of effluent from the stoma appliance can lead to significant skin irritation. This can cause further difficulty in keeping the appliance appropriately placed, setting the stage for a vicious cycle. This can be prevented, or at least minimized by appropriate preoperative siting of the stoma.

Retraction

This can occur in the early or late phase and may also lead to seepage of effluent setting off the vicious cycle of skin excoriation. In mildly symptomatic patients, a convex appliance may be useful to decrease bowel leakage. For severe conditions, a local revision or a relocation of the stoma may be required.

Late complications occur more than 30 days after surgery and include parastomal hernia, prolapse, retraction, stenosis, parastomal skin lesions, and alterations in quality of life.

Parastomal Hernia

This is a leading long-term complication seen in end stomas. The prophylactic use of synthetic mesh in the initial stoma creation has been of recent interest [6, 18]. Conservative measures for management include weight loss, exercise, and the use of a hernia belt. Surgical repair is solely indicated for symptomatic patients or those with emergent presentations. Further details on this topic are discussed in Chap. 13.

Prolapse

A prolapsing stoma can lead to a poorly fitting appliance and subsequent trauma to the mucosa, causing ulceration and bleeding. A conservative approach is initially adopted for this complication with frequent manual reduction. For a temporary ileostomy that has fulfilled its objective, a reversal serves as a definitive treatment. Local procedures for treatment are akin to Delorme's and Altemeir, frequently used in rectal prolapse [19].

Stomal Stenosis/Stricture

Stomal stenosis is usually preceded by vascular compromise in the early postoperative period. Conservative treatment of a stenosis within the subcutaneous layer is typically with mechanical dilation. A revision may be required if local dilation fails.

Parastomal Skin Conditions

The moist skin around the stoma is a favorable environment for candida infection. This can be treated with anti-fungal powder. Dermatitis of peristomal skin may result from a reaction to irritating bowel content or an allergy to material(s) in the appliance. Parastomal skin complications include allergic and non-allergic dermatitis [4]. Inflammatory bowel disease patients may develop pyoderma gangrenosum.

Altered Quality of Life

Ideally, all patients who have an ileostomy should have access to an ostomy nurse for follow-up care. Access to these specialty care nurses can significantly decrease the leakage rate, skin problems, and the use of accessories. Additionally, quality-of-life scores have been shown to improve with these services [4].

Ileostomy Reversal

Temporary ileostomy creation implies the need for a second surgery to reestablish intestinal continuity. There is no absolute consensus as to the timing of the closure of loop ileostomies, but in many centers, this is done roughly 2–3 months after the primary surgery [20, 21]. Early closure of DLI after proctectomy might entail a higher risk of AL, particularly if early closure was done within 2 weeks of DLI formation [22].

References

1. Rowe KM, Schiller LR. Ileostomy diarrhea: pathophysiology and management. Proc (Bayl Univ Med Cent). 2020;33:218–26.
2. Martin ST, Vogel JD. Intestinal stomas indications, management, and complications. Adv Surg. 2012;46:19–49.
3. Montedori A, Cirocchi R, Farinella E, Sciannameo F, Abraha I. Covering ileo- or colostomy in anterior resection for rectal carcinoma. Cochrane Database of Syst Rev. 2010;5:CD006878.
4. Husain SG, Cataldo TE. Late stomal complications. Clin Colon Rectal Surg. 2008;21(1):31–40.
5. Güenaga KF, Lustosa SAS, Saad SS, Saconato H, Matos D. Ileostomy or colostomy for temporary decompression of colorectal anastomosis. Cochrane Database Syst Rev. 2007;2007:CD004647.
6. Hendren S, Hammond K, Glasgow SC, Perry WB, Buie WD, Steele SR, Rafferty J. Clinical practice guidelines for ostomy surgery. Dis Colon Rectum. 2015;58(4):375–87.
7. Manzenreiter L, Spaun G, Weitzendorfer M, Luketina R, Antoniou SA, Wundsam H, Koch OO, Emmanuel K. A proposal for a tailored approach to diverting ostomy for colorectal anastomosis. Minerva Chir. 2018;73(1):29–35.
8. Chen J, Wang DR, Zhang JR, Li P, Niu G, Lu Q. Meta-analysis of temporary ileostomy versus colostomy for colorectal anastomoses. Acta Chir Belg. 2013;113(5):330–9.
9. Balla A, Saraceno F, Rullo M, Morales-Conde S, Targarona Soler EM, Di Saverio S, et al. Protective ileostomy creation after anterior resection of the rectum: shared decision-making or still subjective? Color Dis. 2023;25(4):647–59.
10. Danielsen AK, Burcharth J, Rosenberg J. Patient education has a positive effect in patients with a stoma: a systematic review. Color Dis. 2013;15(6):e276–83.
11. Kumar A, Daga R, Vijayaragaran P, Prakash A, Singh RK, Behari E, et al. Anterior resection for rectal carcinoma-risk factors for anastomotic leaks and strictures. World J Gastroenterol. 2011;17:1475–9.
12. Bax TW, McNevin MS. The value of diverting loop ileostomy on the high-risk colon and rectal anastomosis. Am J Surg. 2007;193:585–7.
13. Gessler B, Haglid E, Angete E. Loop ileostomies in colorectal cancer patients-morbidity and risk factors for non-reversal. J Surg Res. 2012;178:708–14.
14. Liu J, Bruch HP, Farke S, Nolde J, Schwandner O. Stoma formation for fecal diversion: a plea for the laparoscopic approach. Tech Coloproctol. 2005;9(1):9–14.
15. Franklyn J, Varghese G, Mittal R, Rebekah G, Jesudason MR, Perakath B. A prospective randomized controlled trial comparing early postoperative complications in patients undergoing loop colostomy with and without a stoma rod. Color Dis. 2017;19(7):675–80.
16. Erwin-Toth P, Thompson SJ, Davis JS, Erwin-Toth P, Thompson SJ, Davis JS. Factors impacting the quality of life of people with an ostomy in North America: results from the dialogue study. J Wound Ostomy Continence Nurse. 2012;39:417–22.
17. Kann BR. Early stomal complications. Clin Colon Rectal Surg. 2008;21(1):23–30.
18. Jones HG, Rees M, Aboumarzouk OM, et al. Prosthetic mesh placement for the prevention of parastomal herniation. Cochrane Database Syst Rev. 2018;7:CD008905.
19. Tsujinaka S, Tan KY, Miyakura Y, Fukano R, Oshima M, Konishi F, Rikiyama T. Current management of intestinal stomas and their complications. J Anus Rectum Colon. 2020;4(1):25–33.
20. Gustafsson CP, Gunnarsson U, Dahlstrand U, Lindforss U. Loop ileostomy reversal-patient-related characteristics influencing time to closure. Int J Colorectal Dis. 2018;33:593–600.

21. Platell C, Barwood N, Makin G. Clinical utility of a de-functioning loop ileostomy. ANZ J Surg. 2005;75:147–51.
22. Emile SH, Horesh N, Garoufalia Z, Gefen R, Ray-Offor E, Wexner SD. Outcomes of early versus standard closure of diverting ileostomy after proctectomy: meta-analysis and meta-regression analysis of randomized controlled trials. Ann Surg. 2023;279:613–9. https://doi.org/10.1097/SLA.0000000000006109. Epub ahead of print. PMID: 37788345.

# Chapter 2
Laparoscopic Colostomy

Emeka Ray-Offor, Elisa Cassinotti, Ludovica Baldari, and Luigi Boni

Introduction

Over the centuries, the practice of surgical diversion has evolved in different specialties of surgery. A stoma is a surgical creation involving the exteriorization of a hollow viscus (airway, urinary, or gastrointestinal tract) to the outside of the body. Specifically in colorectal surgery, a purposeful anastomosis between a segment of the colon and the skin is termed a colostomy. Historically, successful decompression procedures of the colon in the latter half of the mid-eighteenth century by Drs. M. Pillore, C. Duret, and subsequently other surgeons were for advanced malignant obstructions, the worst cases of injury, or disease of the colon or rectum [1]. These procedures invariably were accompanied by a high incidence of mortality; hence, colostomy creation was conservatively practiced. An evolution of the practice of colostomy came through the high case volume from the military experience of World War II, demonstrating its efficacy with a striking decrease in mortality rates [2, 3]. The exteriorization of the colon with colostomy has become more frequently

E. Ray-Offor (✉)
College of Health Sciences, University of Port Harcourt, Choba, Rivers State, Nigeria

Colorectal/Minimal Access Surgery Unit, Department of Surgery, University of Port Harcourt Teaching Hospital, Port Harcourt, Rivers State, Nigeria
e-mail: emeka.ray-offor@uniport.edu.ng

E. Cassinotti · L. Boni
University of Milan, Milan, Italy

General and Minimally Invasive Surgery, Fondazione IRCCS—Ca' Granda—Ospedale Maggiore, Policlinico di Milano, Milan, Italy

L. Baldari
General and Minimally Invasive Surgery, Fondazione IRCCS—Ca' Granda—Ospedale Maggiore, Policlinico di Milano, Milan, Italy

© The Author(s), under exclusive license to Springer Nature Switzerland AG 2024
E. Ray-Offor, R. J. Rosenthal (eds.), *Colorectal & Hernia Laparoscopic Surgery*, https://doi.org/10.1007/978-3-031-63490-1_2

used in colorectal surgery when indicated, being created in an elective or emergency setting.

In the late twentieth century, we witnessed the advent of laparoscopic surgery, with wide applications in the management of surgical diseases. A laparoscopic approach to stoma creation has increasingly been practiced. Some advantages of this technique include a panoramic view of the abdominal cavity, a lower postoperative analgesia requirement, an earlier time to return to bowel function, earlier tolerance of a solid diet, and fewer postoperative complications. Laparoscopic colostomy may be temporary, thereby offering a chance for definitive treatment of the underlying pathology, hence requiring a second operation for closure. Alternatively, it can be a permanent stoma, usually created with the entire luminal circumference of the bowel as an end stoma. An end colostomy is usually sited in the left iliac fossa, whereas a temporary transverse colostomy is brought out in the right hypochondrium, and the effluent is solid. It is noteworthy that about half of the patients who undergo surgical resection with stoma creation deemed temporary are never reversed [4, 5]. This underscores the significance of the decision to create a stoma as nontrivial and can have a significant effect on patients' livelihood. Some key considerations are related to the indication, type, site, technique, and duration of creation.

In all, proper management of the stoma involves preoperative patient education, counseling, and skin marking, with adequate postoperative follow-up mitigating significant morbidities [6].

Relevant Anatomy

The large intestine is a hollow viscus and part of the gastrointestinal system with a variable length of about 150 cm, referred to as the colon. Three distinctive features of the colon are the non-mesenteric fat pads on its serosal surface (appendices epiploicae), three thickened bands of the outer longitudinal muscle of the colon wall (taenia coli), and outpouchings of this wall between the taenia (haustra).

The colon comprises different segments. Proximally, the cecum is entirely covered by the visceral peritoneum, terminating posterior-medially in the ileocecal valve (ICV). Of note is that the competence of ICV in the setting of colon obstruction leads to a closed-loop obstruction. A vestigial appendix is located at the base of the cecum with a slit-like opening. The straight, continuing ascending colon is between the cecum and the hepatic flexure, covered on its anterior surface by the visceral peritoneum, while its posterior surface is fused with the retroperitoneum. Its lateral peritoneal reflection forms a thickened line (white line of Toldt), which is a helpful guide for the mobilization of the ascending colon.

The next segment is the longest and traverses the abdomen from the hepatic flexure to the splenic flexure. This transverse colon is entirely covered by the visceral peritoneum and attached to the posterior abdominal wall by a mesocolon. The descending colon continues inferiorly from the splenic flexure and, like the ascending colon, is covered on its anterior and lateral surfaces and lateral peritoneal reflection (white line of Toldt)—a landmark for left colon mobilization. The sigmoid colon connects the descending colon to the rectum, and like the transverse colon, is entirely covered by visceral peritoneum. Fusion of the taenia coli marks the transition from the sigmoid colon to the rectum.

Colon segments with mesentery afford the mobility needed for stoma creation. This fact naturally selects the sites for colostomy as the transverse colon (transverse colostomy), the sigmoid colon (sigmoid colostomy), or the intraperitoneal cecum (caecostomy). However, any other segment of the colon may be mobilized to create a stoma, ensuring it meets the underlying stoma creation principles of protruding, tension-free, and well vascularized.

Colostomies can be classified based on the portion of the colon lumen connected to the skin—the connection of the entire luminal circumference to the skin, an end colostomy, or part of the bowel to form a loop colostomy. Based on the type of configuration of the stoma, a double barrel colostomy, as the name implies, has two end circumferences of the colon, apposed, and the colon attached to the skin. Complete isolation of openings in the proximal and distal segments (Devine colostomy) will prevent the spillage of feces into the distal opening, which now becomes a mucous fistula [7].

Indications

1. Protecting low pelvic anastomosis
   An ostomy is considered for a pelvic anastomosis <5 to 6 cm, including coloanal anastomosis. The impact of pelvic sepsis and reoperation rates is certainly reduced with this diversion. However, based on considerable quality-of-life implications, the decision to proceed with a stoma should be a highly individualized one, taking into account both the negative impact on role and function and balanced with the benefits of leak risk reduction [8, 9]. The demonstrated risk factors for leak complications include male gender, anastomotic height, obesity, steroid use, malnutrition, steroid use, and prior irradiation [10, 11].
2. Diverting acute traumatic injury to the colon
   The creation of a defunctioning stoma for anorectal disease in patients in whom no resection or anastomosis is required appears eminently suited for laparoscopic techniques. This creation in traumatic injury of the colon is to avoid or minimize intraperitoneal contamination.
3. Bowel defunctionalization from distal obstruction
   A diversion by a colostomy can be created to achieve decompression arising from a distal bowel obstruction to prevent perforation with ensuing abdominal contamination. Diverting colostomy can be used as a bridge to primary resection in the setting of an obstructing malignancy, allowing the dilated proximal bowel to regain normal caliber and be optimized for subsequent anastomosis. The treatment of distal colonic malignancy may involve a diversion followed by primary

resection (staged surgery). An end colostomy is part of Hartmann procedure and abdominoperineal resection for low rectal and/or anal carcinoma.
4. Diverting a distal chronically benign pathology

   Complex fistulas like entero-urethral, vesical, or vaginal may require a diverting stoma. The ongoing fecal insult that mitigates resolution is diverted. Radiation proctitis and perianal sepsis are other indications for fecal diversion by laparoscopic colostomy. In severe perianal Crohn's disease, surgeons prefer a loop colostomy instead of an ileostomy in patients with preexisting renal insufficiency. Generally, colostomy is considered over ileostomy in those in whom stoma reversal is unlikely due to a higher risk of dehydration and electrolyte abnormalities associated with permanent ileostomy."

Contraindications

An absolute contraindication to laparoscopic colostomy is in hemodynamically unstable patients. Such patients may not withstand the physiological changes associated with pneumoperitoneum and the trauma of the procedure. Additionally, a tensely distended abdomen from complete bowel obstruction is unsuitable for this laparoscopic approach. The reason is the loss of domain for pneumoperitoneum and poor visualization of intended colon segments for stoma creation resulting from the distended bowels. The heightened risk of iatrogenic bowel injury can lead to catastrophic peritoneal contamination. In this setting, an open colostomy is advised with an initial decompression of the colon upon gaining peritoneal access.

Relative contraindication to laparoscopic colostomy includes a history of multiple abdominal surgeries and multiple adhesions associated with a high risk of iatrogenic injury. A surgeon's expertise is also a limiting consideration; hence, a critical self-audit is required before undertaking laparoscopic intervention.

Preoperative Preparation

A full clinical assessment for general anesthesia is necessary with routine complete blood count, chemistry, and cardiothoracic evaluation. Informed consent is obtained. Structured patient education for patients' psychosocial needs is reported to have a positive effect on the quality of life as well as on cost [6]. An ostomy nurse specialist is helpful for patient education, consenting, and skin marking of colostomy patients, especially in an elective setting. The selection of the stoma site requires careful consideration of the body habitus of the patient and an assessment in sitting, standing, and supine positions. A surrounding 2-inch flat area of healthy skin around the marked site ensures an adequate appliance seal. Consequently, the stoma site should be remote from bony prominences, planned incisions, old incisions, and skin creases. It is preferable to site the stoma at the apex of a fat mound, where possible, in obese patients for effective self-care post-creation. Also, multiple sites should be marked in patients with obesity, difficult anatomy (prior scars), and where operative plans are not certain.

Prophylactic antibiotics administration (oral and intravenous) and bowel preparation when feasible are instituted before surgery according to the hospital protocol. The basic operating room laparoscopic equipment comprises a 10 mm 30-degree laparoscope, two 10 mm trocars, and an additional 5 mm trocar, 10 mm Babcock forceps, Yohan atraumatic forceps, and an energy device.

Technique

Adequate induction of general endotracheal anesthesia is performed. The patient is carefully positioned in the supine or modified lithotomy position with stirrups. Precautionary measures include careful padding and protection of all areas of potential pressure injury. The abdomen, pelvis, and perineum are prepped and draped in the usual sterile manner. An infra- or supra-umbilical vertical incision is made through which a 10 mm Hasson cannula is carefully placed. Carbon dioxide pneumoperitoneum of 12–15 mmHg is achieved. A second 10 mm cannula is carefully placed under direct vision through a horizontal stab wound in the previously identified left iliac fossa colostomy site for sigmoid colostomy. A diagnostic laparoscopy is performed, and the colon segment for exteriorization is identified. With the 10 mm diameter Babcock or the Yohan atraumatic grasping forceps, a loop of the distal sigmoid colon, which would easily reach above the skin level in a tension-free manner, is isolated and carefully maintained in its appropriate anatomic orientation (Fig. 2.1).

The colostomy site is then developed by excising a 2 cm disk of skin and incising the underlying fat and anterior rectus sheath in a cephalad to caudad direction. The rectus fibers are spread along their axis. The posterior sheath and peritoneum are

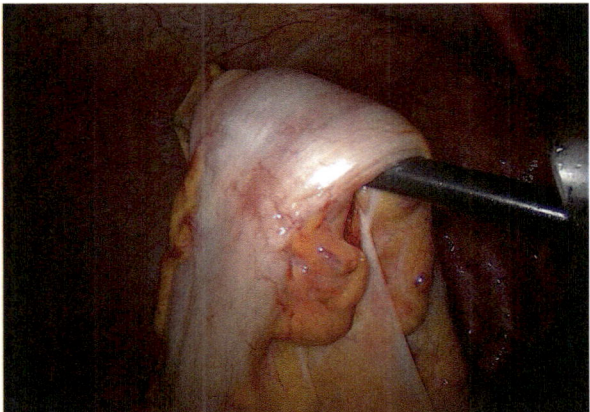

Fig. 2.1 Mobilising bowel segment for loop colostomy

incised in the cephalad to caudad direction. For a loop colostomy, the loop of the colon is delivered through the stoma site, such that 5 cm rests above the skin in a tension-free manner.

In some instances, a rod is placed under the mesenteric margin and sutured in place with 2-0 silk. The abdomen is desufflated as the umbilical port site is closed. The colostomy is then matured by incising with electrocautery, flush on the efferent limb. A 3-0 chromic maturation suture is utilized, taking full-thickness bites of the cut edge, seromuscular bites at the skin level, and intracuticular bites of the skin. A loop colostomy is formed (Fig. 2.2).

A stoma appliance is placed over the healthy, pink, well-everted stoma. The patient is discharged to the recovery room in stable condition.

For an end colostomy, a transected stapled end of the proximal colon is delivered through the stoma site. The stapled bowel end is then excised, and the exteriorized bowel is fixed to the skin with an interrupted absorbable 2.0 suture. This is preceded by anchoring sutures to the superficial fascia of the anterior abdominal wall. (Fig. 2.3).

A colostomy is usually functional within 72 hours of surgery. A daily inspection of the colostomy is easily done by the preferred use of a transparent appliance over the stoma at operation. Early complications of bleeding or mucosal separation are resolved by adding hemostatic or reapproximating sutures. Simple debridement may resolve partial ischemic necrosis after assessing the adequacy of the aperture. Other possible complications are early stenosis or retraction and contact dermatitis of the surrounding skin. For defunctioning colostomy, patients are subsequently worked up for definitive treatment on an outpatient or inpatient basis. A detailed discussion on the care of the ostomy is beyond the scope of this chapter. Stoma nurse therapists and ostomy support groups are beneficial [6].

Suffice it to note that the colostomy may need to be refashioned in the theatre. A range of long-term complications associated with colostomy includes parastomal

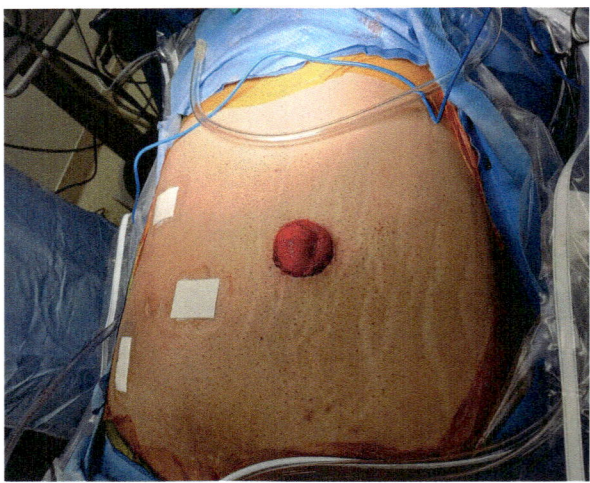

Fig. 2.2 Loop colostomy on the left side of the abdomen

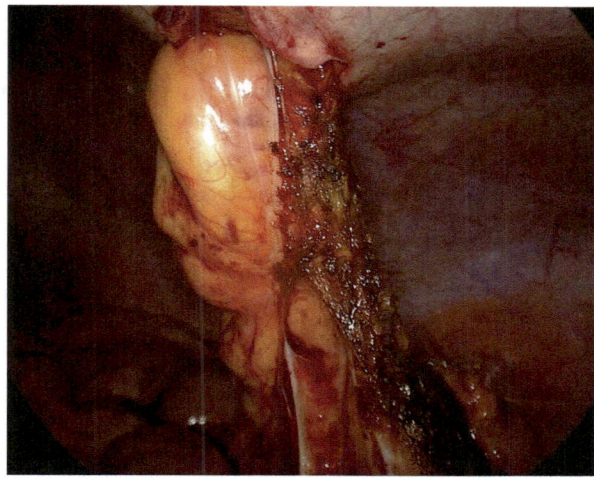

Fig. 2.3 Delivery of colon for end colostomy through stoma site on the left abdominal wall

hernia, prolapse, peristomal pyoderma gangrenosum, obstruction, and depression [12]. There is no universally accepted time for stoma reversal, but generally, this is performed from 6 to 8 weeks post-primary surgery. A water-soluble contrast radiology study ought to be performed before the reestablishment of gut continuity.

Special Notes

The complications of stoma prolapse/retraction, parastomal hernia, surgical site infection (SSI), and incisional hernias are higher following laparoscopic colostomy than laparoscopic ileostomy [13, 14]. For the prevention of parastomal hernias, randomized controlled trials have demonstrated significantly lower rates of parastomal hernia occurrence when synthetic mesh was placed at the time of stoma creation [15, 16]. Laparoscopic permanent sigmoid stoma creation through the extraperitoneal route may take a little more time compared with the transperitoneal colostomy, but this route may reduce the incidence of parastomal hernia [17].

References

1. Poer DH. The place of colostomy in present-day surgery. South Surg. 1948;14(2):130–42.
2. Plasencia A, Bahna H. Diverting ostomy: for whom, when, what, where and why. Clin Colon Rectal Surg. 2019;32(3):171–5.
3. Young CJ, Eyers AA, Solomon MJ. Defunctioning of the anorectum: historical controlled study of laparoscopic vs. open procedures. Dis Colon Rectum. 1998;41:190–4.

4. Vermeulen J, Gosselink MP, Busschbach JJ, Lange JF. Avoiding or reversing Hartmann's procedure provides improved quality of life after perforated diverticulitis. J Gastrointest Surg. 2010;14(4):651–7.
5. Roig JV, Cantos M, Balciscueta Z, et al.; Sociedad Valenciana de Cirugía Cooperative Group. Hartmann's operation: how often is it reversed and at what cost? A multicentre study. Color Dis. 2011;13(12):e396–e402.
6. Danielsen AK, Burcharth J, Rosenberg J. Patient education has a positive effect in patients with a stoma: a systematic review. Color Dis. 2013;15(6):e276–83.
7. Ochsner A, DeBakey M, Rothschild J. The "defunctionalizing" colostomy (devine): a rational preparatory procedure for resection of lesions of the large bowel. JAMA. 1939;113(7):568–73.
8. Shimizu H, Yamaguchi S, Ishii T, Kondo H, Hara K, Takemoto K, et al. Who needs diverting ileostomy following laparoscopic low anterior resection in rectal cancer patients? Analysis of 417 patients in a single institute. Surg Endosc. 2020;34(2):839–46.
9. Phan K, Oh L, Ctercteko G, Pathma-Nathan N, El Khoury T, Azam H, et al. Does a stoma reduce the risk of anastomotic leak and need for re-operation following low anterior resection for rectal cancer: systematic review and meta-analysis of randomized controlled trials. J Gastrointest Oncol. 2019;10(2):179–87.
10. Mäkelä JT, Kiviniemi H, Laitinen S. Risk factors for anastomotic leakage after left-sided colorectal resection with rectal anastomosis. Dis Colon Rectum. 2003;46:653–60.
11. Lee WS, Yun SH, Roh YN, et al. Risk factors and clinical outcome for anastomotic leakage after total mesorectal excision for rectal cancer. World J Surg. 2008;32:1124–9.
12. Du R, Zhou J, Tong G, Chang Y, Li D, Wang F, Ding X, Zhang Q, Wang W, Wang L, Wang D. Postoperative morbidity and mortality after anterior resection with preventive diverting loop ileostomy versus loop colostomy for rectal cancer: a updated systematic review and meta-analysis. Eur J Surg Oncol. 2021;47(7):1514–25.
13. Jänes A, Cengiz Y, Israelsson LA. Preventing parastomal hernia with a prosthetic mesh: a 5-year follow-up of a randomized study. World J Surg. 2009;33:118–21.
14. Jänes A, Cengiz Y, Israelsson LA. Randomized clinical trial of the use of a prosthetic mesh to prevent parastomal hernia. Br J Surg. 2004;91:280–2.
15. López-Cano M, Lozoya-Trujillo R, Quiroga S, Sánchez JL, Vallribera F, Martí M, et al. Use of a prosthetic mesh to prevent parastomal hernia during laparoscopic abdominoperineal resection: a randomized controlled trial. Hernia. 2012;16:661–7.
16. Serra-Aracil X, Bombardo-Junca J, Moreno-Matias J, Darnell A, Mora-Lopez L, Alcantara-Moral M, et al. Randomized, controlled, prospective trial of the use of a mesh to prevent parastomal hernia. Ann Surg. 2009;249:583–7.
17. Wang FB, Pu YW, Zhong FY, Lv XD, Yang ZX, Xing CG. Laparoscopic permanent sigmoid stoma creation through the extraperitoneal route versus transperitoneal route. A meta-analysis of stoma-related complications. Saudi Med J. 2015;36(2):159–63.

Chapter 3
Laparoscopic Colectomy

Olusegun Komolafe

Introduction

Laparoscopic colectomy (LC) was first reported in 1991 [1, 2]. Early randomized controlled trials (RCTs) demonstrated equivalence with open resections and confirmed other intuitive benefits: shorter length of stay, and less analgesic requirements [3–5]. Some studies found improved oncological outcomes for patients having laparoscopic colonic resections [6, 7]. LC is now accepted as the default procedure, recommended by national and regional colorectal societies, provided surgeons are adequately skilled and have the necessary equipment available. The conversation has moved from whether LC is safe or appropriate, to ensuring that surgeons are adequately trained to become competent at laparoscopic colonic resection. It should be noted that inclusion criteria for the landmark RCTs were patients having segmental right, left, and sigmoid colectomies. Patients needing transverse colectomy, or any rectal resection, were excluded. The outcomes for segmental LC have been extrapolated to the more technically challenging transverse colectomy, with subsequent studies supporting this [8]. The evidence for, and practice of, minimally invasive surgery for rectal pathology is varied and nuanced, well beyond the scope of this chapter (Part II).

There is debate about what constitutes a laparoscopic vs a laparoscopic-assisted vs an open colonic resection. The Lanarkshire definition is simple and widely applicable. If the tumor segment is mobilized laparoscopically AND the relevant vessels are divided laparoscopically, that is a laparoscopic procedure, regardless of whether the anastomosis is fashioned intra- or extra-corporeal, laparoscopically, or manually. If EITHER the tumor segment is mobilized laparoscopically OR the vessels are divided laparoscopically, but both are not completed laparoscopically, that is a

---

O. Komolafe (✉)
University Hospital Wishaw, Wishaw, Scotland

University of Glasgow, Glasgow, Scotland
e-mail: segun.komolafe@lanarkshire.scot.nhs.uk

© The Author(s), under exclusive license to Springer Nature
Switzerland AG 2024
E. Ray-Offor, R. J. Rosenthal (eds.), *Colorectal & Hernia Laparoscopic Surgery*, https://doi.org/10.1007/978-3-031-63490-1_3

laparoscopic-assisted procedure. If any incision is made PRIOR to both tumor mobilization and vessel division, which are then completed through the incision, that is an open procedure, regardless of whether that is how the operation was commenced. It cannot be overstated that conversion to open surgery is not a failure of technique and sometimes is the correct course of action.

Relevant Anatomy

Appreciation of the embryological development of the midgut and hindgut helps inform LC. Before rotation *in utero*, the gut and mesentery are midline structures. Mobilizing the colon is restoring it to the original embryological midline location. Correct surgical dissection follows embryological planes of cleavage. Coupled with this must be an appreciation of the blood supply and lymphatic drainage of different parts of the colon, with anatomical variants. An elegant review article by Mike and Kano lays out useful anatomical considerations related to the colonic blood supply and lymphatic drainage to guide appropriate segmental resection [9].

There are specific considerations in LC, for surgeons transitioning from open surgery, or those expanding their laparoscopic skills. The complexity of colonic resection sets it apart from procedures like appendicectomy or cholecystectomy: there is a need to operate in more than one abdominal quadrant, and to securely ligate named vessels. The general convention for mobilizing the colon laparoscopically, especially for malignant disease, is "medial to lateral", incising the visceral peritoneum to open up the embryological plane between the mesocolon, and the true retroperitoneum. This differs from the convention at open surgery of mobilizing the colon of the parietes, along the white line of Toldt, in a lateral to medial direction.

It should be borne in mind that the thin patient can be technically as challenging as the obese patient. A thin patient will not have much fat to help delineate anatomic planes, and it can be very difficult to identify avascular embryological planes, and not stray out of them. The obese patient is challenging, on various counts: it can be difficult to get access into the abdomen; they are more difficult to ventilate; it is harder to maintain a clear view intra-operatively; and mesocolic fat tends to be friable, fracturing easily, making traction difficult. It is informative that patients with a high BMI were not included in the landmark RCTs.

Indications/Contra-indications

It is now accepted that patients with cancer, or complex, chronic disease should be managed under the umbrella of a multi-disciplinary team (MDT) [10]. A colorectal cancer MDT will typically consist of an MDT administrator, colorectal cancer nurse specialist, stoma therapy nurse, radiologist, clinical oncologist, medical oncologist, histopathologist, palliative physician, and surgeon. In resource-limited environments of some low and middle-income countries (LMICs), this may not be achievable, however, the mindset of teamwork, and developing pathways, to manage patients requiring colonic resections in a manner that is consistent and systematized can only improve outcomes. A good MDT process is one where there is a cross-specialty discussion of each patient's unique case, on its own merits, the patient's investigations are reviewed, scientific evidence and guidelines are considered, then optimal management is determined by consensus, bespoke to that patient.

In the absence of a functioning MDT, surgeons must be aware of the current evidence base, and guidelines, to present the best options to the patient, arriving at a management plan as equal partners with the patient. This is particularly relevant for emergent cases, where patients have not been fully staged, and the surgeon may have to make crucial judgment calls peri-operatively. The days of the "Lone Ranger" surgeon, single-handedly deciding the best treatment or operation for a patient must be consigned to the past [11, 12]. Similarly, there needs to be a paradigm shift in cultures where the oldest, senior surgeon is deferred to when it comes to decision-making, with a commitment to evidence-based practice, and flattened hierarchy with genuine teamwork, to ensure better outcomes for patients [13].

Many single-handed surgeons around the globe routinely link up with other surgeons, and surgical departments, through the Internet, for MDT meetings, mentorship, and peer support. This is an area that surgeons in LMICs may want to explore and expand further, especially if practicing in isolated, remote regions. One of the benefits of the COVID-19 pandemic is the wider acceptance of online teamwork and decision-making.

A surgeon must be proficient in laparoscopic resection, or have appropriate supervision, before undertaking LC. Oncological sanctity must never be compromised; and it is at best negligent, if not downright criminal, to be "practicing" on patients. The resections performed in the landmark RCTs are procedures appropriate for surgeons new to LC: right hemicolectomy, and sigmoid colectomy, ideally in average-sized patients, with virgin abdomens.

Pre-operative Preparation

The patient should have appropriate cross-sectional imaging. It is worthwhile for surgeons to develop the ability to assess CT images for themselves, to differentiate between normal anatomy and pathology. A surgeon well-versed with CT images can glean important information including anatomical variants in the named vessels; the location of the target pathology, especially relevant if the surgeon did not colonoscope the patient; redundancy of bowel loops, involvement of adjacent organs, etc. This is particularly pertinent in healthcare systems where reporting of CT scans is not standardized, nor regulated, so may lack quality, detail, and accuracy.

It is possible to perform LC with simple monopolar or bipolar diathermy, however, advanced energy devices are better at hemostasis, and facilitating dissection. In simplest terms, these devices generate energy in one of two ways: by passing a current between the jaws, essentially modified bipolar diathermy, (Ligasure®, ENSEAL®, Caiman®, Voyant®); or, by high-frequency vibration of one of the jaws (Harmonic Ace®). Some devices are a combination of both modalities of energy generation (THUNDERBEAT®). The basics of laparoscopic setup, including energy devices, have been covered previously [see Principles and Practice of Laparoscopic Surgery volume 1, Chaps. 2 and 3].

Anesthesia

Enhanced Recovery After Surgery (ERAS) principles are widely accepted with various templates and pathways widely available for adoption and modification in individual units. The details are beyond the scope of this chapter, but surgical teams and systems should seek to adopt ERAS principles [14, 15]. This involves every stage of a patient's journey of care from pre-habilitation once the diagnosis is confirmed to peri-operative care, including standardized multi-modal anesthesia then post-op protocolized care with specific ERAS targets based on clear scientific evidence.

The modern-day surgeon must be rigorous in the application of scientific evidence to his/her practice, rather than anecdotal evidence, or "what we always do". A good ERAS pathway will protocolize the majority of a patient's journey of care, along with evidence-based principles, to improve outcomes. A permanent member of the department should ideally be given responsibility for this, in many cases, a dedicated senior nurse or physician's assistant can help coordinate an ERAS pathway, as well as audit adherence and outcomes.

General Principles

- Tumour location must be clearly defined before surgery such as tattooing just distal to the tumor site with methylene blue dye at the time of diagnostic colonoscopy as there is no facility to palpate the lesion at laparoscopic dissection.
- Lesions that are small or posterior may be imperceptible laparoscopically. If the lesion has been tattooed, the surgeon must know the tattooed location of the tumor. Except for lesions in the caecal pole or close to the ileocaecal valve, the author's practice is to tattoo distal to all lesions, on two different sides at the same distance from the tumor. For lesions in the rectum or sigmoid, the tattoo is injected 10–20 mm from the distal edge of the tumor. Experienced Radiology input at MDT also helps with accurate tumor localization.
- Avoid grasping the bowel as much as possible: retract epiploic appendages, pericolic fat, mesocolon, and small bowel mesentery preferentially. Obese patients have fat that is friable, and fractures easily, so in certain scenarios, judicious

handling of the bowel with an atraumatic grasper is necessary. In this scenario, a broad/wide grip spreads the force, rather than a pinch, or small grip.
- Surgeons must be completely conversant with their energy devices, this is non-negotiable. Most energy devices can safely divide vessels up to 7 mm so are adequate for sealing the mesenteric vessels, using a "double-burn" technique: traction on the vessel is relaxed, then the vessel is sealed twice, a millimeter or two apart, with the division of the vessel at the seal nearer the bowel, that way ensuring the residual stump is doubly sealed. It might be prudent in certain situations to use a clipping device such as Hem-o-lok®, Ligaclip®, or Ligamax® to ensure that the vessels are secured safely before division.
- The more "important" hand is the non-dominant hand, which maintains traction. The retracting hand does the majority of the work, displaying the bowel or mesentery for the operating hand to then divide, dissect, etc. Aim to develop a 1–2–3 tactic; for example 1–the mesocolon is stretched–2–the energy device starts to divide–3–whilst this is happening, the retracting hand is moved along to establish traction in the next area to be divided, so there is constant sequential progress and surgical efficiency.
- For LC where the pelvis is not entered, the urinary catheter can be taken out at the end of the procedure. There is no need to routinely leave a catheter without patient-specific, or case-specific indications. Similarly, drains should only be inserted judiciously, for specific reasons, such as drainage of an "oozy" procedure, or to drain lavage fluid for 12–24 h only. Drains do NOT prevent anastomotic leaks, nor septic complications, and are a major cause of post-operative pain, impeding patient mobility and recovery.

Right Hemicolectomy

The patient is placed in a supine position, with both arms tucked into the body. Entry into the abdomen and establishment of pneumo-peritoneum is by whichever method a surgeon is most familiar with. Open cutdown with the Hasson technique, inserting a blunt port for the camera, is widely considered safe [16]. This author's preference is to cut down on the right or left SIDE of the umbilicus, on the OPPOSITE side of where the stoma would be brought out in the case of an anastomotic leak—somewhat pessimistically! A 12 mm curvilinear cutdown beside the umbilicus can easily be extended in either direction by 1–2 cm to allow specimen extraction, avoiding having to make another incision (Fig. 3.1). Two working 5 mm ports are inserted under vision on the left side of the abdomen. A further fourth port can be inserted on the right side if further traction is needed.

The essential steps of laparoscopic right hemicolectomy are

1. Omentum and transverse colon placed cephalad above the liver, then patient placed in head down position. The small bowel retracted towards the left side, then a lateral tilt is performed so the right side is upwards, and the small bowel

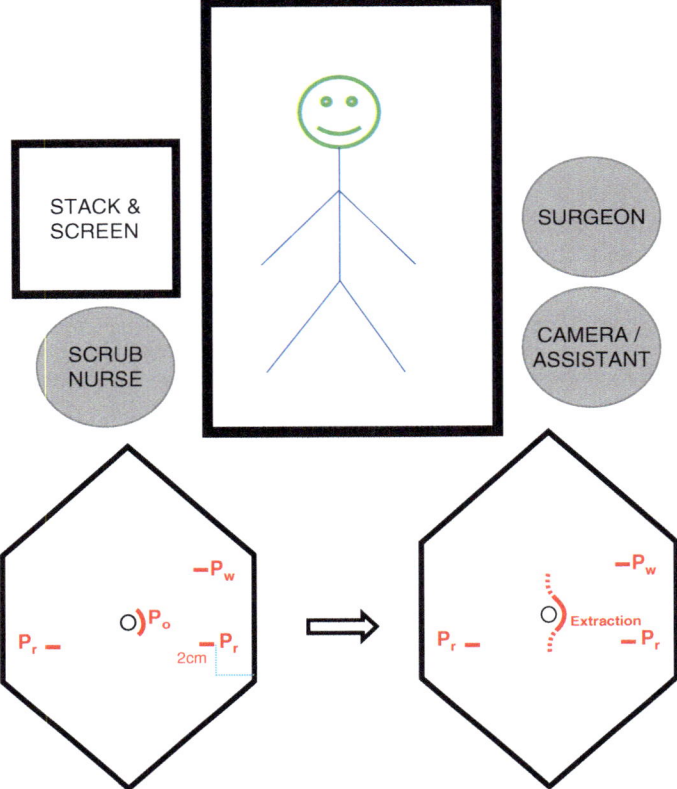

Fig. 3.1 Theatre set up for Lap Right Hemi/Appendicectomy/Ileo-Caecal Resection/Small Bowel Resection. P_o—12 mm Optical Port, P_w—5 mm Working instrument port, P_r—5 mm Retracting instrument port

stays on the left side away from the surgical field. The junction of terminal ileum and caecum is retracted infero-anteriorly using an atraumatic grasper, to stretch out the ileo-colic pedicle, displaying the ileo-caecal junction.

2. The visceral peritoneum is incised in the sulcus posterior to the tented pedicle, to enter the embryological plane between the mesocolon and retroperitoneum. This mainly avascular plane can be developed by blunt dissection laterally towards the posterior aspect of the white line of Toldt. The duodenum should be identified and protected. The retro-colic "cave" can also be developed superomedially to display the third, then second, and first part of the duodenum, cradling the head of the pancreas medially.
3. The line of the pancreas represents a horizon, at which level the ileo-colic vessels, or middle colic vessels, should be divided for cancers of the right or transverse colon respectively. This will ensure a good lymphadenectomy, and at the same time, minimize the risk of injury to the main superior mesenteric vessels.

4. Once the ileocolic vessels have been divided, the mesocolon can be divided in the superior direction towards the medial aspect of the hepatic flexure. The right colic vessels may be encountered in this phase of the dissection and would similarly require ligation close to the root of the mesocolon. This dissection can be taken medially towards the right branch of the middle colic artery. If the tumor is a true right colonic cancer, there is no need to sacrifice the right middle colic artery.
5. The hepatic flexure should be mobilized as this allows full delivery of the right colon for tension-free anastomosis. The colon will remain at this point attached by the gastrocolic momentum, hepato-colic ligaments, and the parieto-colic ligaments along the white line of Toldt. The gastrocolic omentum can be divided, starting at the midline, using the falciform ligament as a landmark. The lesser sac is best entered here, then the gastro-colic omentum divided medial to lateral, to take down the hepato-colic ligament at the flexure. The parietal attachments can be released from the flexure to the caecum, joining up with the previous posterior dissection.
6. Once the cecal pole has been freed, it is important to be careful to dissect the terminal ileum and meso-ileum completely off the pelvic brim, protecting the ureter which runs close at this point. Mobilizing the terminal ileum fully will allow tension-free delivery of the small bowel to facilitate the formation of anastomosis. At this point, the bowel should be fully mobile from the terminal ileum to the proximal transverse colon. Hemostasis and a swab count should be checked. A grasper is secured to the appendix and locked.
7. Attention is then turned towards making an extraction wound by extension of the umbilical cut down. A small 4–5 cm trephine is usually sufficient to deliver the specimen for extra-corporeal anastomosis, after manipulating the appendix into the extraction wound, with the locked grasper. This surgeon's preference at this point is to trim the ileal mesentery close to the ileo-caecal junction and perform a side-to-side stapled ileo-colic anastomosis. The distal colonic division will depend on the tumor location. If there has been obstruction resulting in a thickened, oedematous small bowel, or for high-risk patients such as those with extensive co-morbidities, arteriopathy, or octogenarians, a sutured end-to-end anastomosis is fashioned. Where available, indocyanine green can be infused intravenously, and fluorescence angiography performed to confirm adequate blood supply before bowel division, and before stapling for anastomosis formation (Fig. 3.2).
8. The anastomosis is returned to the abdomen, and the pneumo-peritoneum is re-established using a device such as the Alexis® retractor for maintaining the pneumo-peritoneum. The surgical field is lavaged copiously, hemostasis is confirmed again, and the anastomosis is covered with the omentum. The ports are withdrawn under vision, then the extraction trephine is closed after injection of large volume dilutes local anesthetic into the pre-peritoneal plane on both sides, under direct vision, and the urinary catheter is taken out.

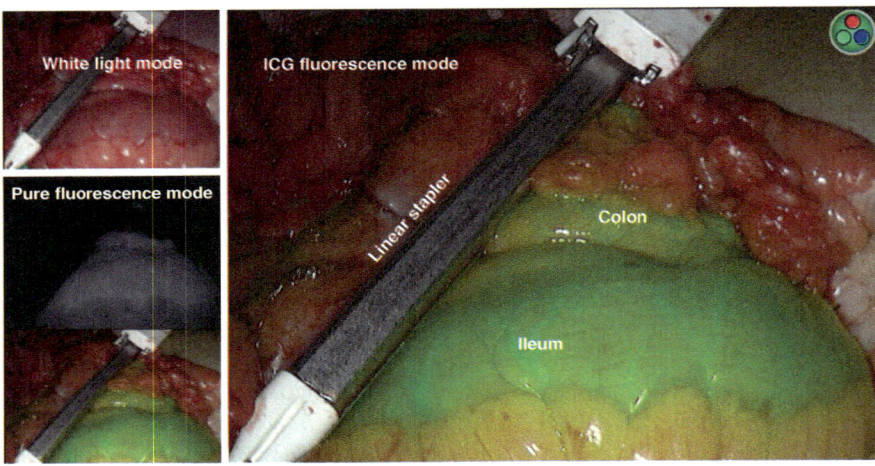

Fig. 3.2 ICG infused during anastomosis of Right Hemicolectomy confirming well-vascularised bowel

Transverse Colectomy

Historically, tumors of the transverse colon have been managed by extended right hemicolectomy, treating the distal midgut as a single anatomical entity. However, this represents a lot of the colon to sacrifice, for example for a mid-transverse colon tumor, supplied by the middle colic pedicle. Equally important are the ileo-caecal valve, and terminal ileum which are routinely sacrificed historically. It is self-evident that if these organs are preserved the patient will have better nutrition, and also gut function, provided oncological sanctity is not compromised [17].

A standard transverse colectomy, taking the middle colic pedicle and nodes, ought to suffice for transverse colon tumors. The crucial technical issue is that both the splenic and hepatic flexures must be fully mobilized to allow tension-free anastomosis. Positioning and access as per right hemicolectomy. A further fourth and fifth port will need to be inserted on the opposite side, to allow taking down both flexures fully.

The essential steps of laparoscopic transverse hemicolectomy are

1. Once pneumo-peritoneum is established, the falciform ligament is divided, to the diaphragm, to allow placement of the greater omentum and transverse colon above the liver, *AFTER* which point the patient is placed in head down position, the entire transverse stretched out, mesocolon stretched cephalad, so middle colic vessels perceptible. The surgeon should be aware while there can be variation in the middle colics, they essentially follow a V or Y configuration, depending on whether the bifurcation is at the mesocolic root, or within the transverse mesocolon.

2. The visceral peritoneum is incised in the sulcus lateral to the tented pedicle, above the "horizon" of the pancreas, and the lesser sac is entered by careful dissection through the mesocolon. The posterior stomach should become apparent at this point. The mesocolon can then safely be divided lateral to the middle colics in both directions, all the way to both flexures.
3. As discussed, the middle colics can then be dissected clearly and divided just above the level of the pancreatic horizon. Once the middle colic vessels have been divided, the lesser sac should be widely open. This medial mesocolic dissection can be taken literally to just above the duodenum on the right, and the tail of the pancreas on the left.
4. Attention should then be turned to taking the colon off the greater omentum. This is best achieved by a combination of inferior traction on the mesocolon and antero-cephalad traction on the greater omentum. As described above, taking the omentum off the colon allows entry into the lesser sac, which has been previously opened from behind the colon, through the mesocolic window. This phase should be initiated in the midline where the lesser sac is most accessible. The gastro-colic ligaments can be fully divided in both directions, all the way around to the hepato-colic ligaments on the right, and lieno-colic ligaments on the left, taking down the hepatic and splenic flexures, respectively.
5. At this point the colon should be fully mobile from the proximal right colon to the distal left colon. A grasper is secured to the colon close to the tumor and locked. The specimen can then be extracted as described above. The anastomosis can be fashioned with a stapler or sutured end to end, and returned to the abdomen, concluding the operation as before.

Left Hemicolectomy

it is crucial to delineate the appropriate oncological procedure for left colon tumors. A left hemicolectomy is for tumors of the proximal left colon, nourished by the left colic pedicle, branching off the inferior mesenteric artery. A distal transverse colon cancer more probably needs a transverse colectomy; and a mid- to distal left colon tumor is more likely to need an "extended" sigmoid colectomy taking the left colic and sigmoid branch of the IMA, sparing the superior haemorrhoidal vessels.

As stated before, an MDT process is crucial, as well as cross-sectional imaging with careful study of the blood supply by the operating surgeon, so he/she is clear pre-operatively what resection/lymphadenectomy is needed, and to consent the patient fully. Position and access are a mirror image of the right hemicolectomy setup (Fig. 3.3), except for a 12 mm working port, to allow insertion of stapler, later on. A fourth port can be inserted on the left side if further traction is needed.

The essential steps of laparoscopic left hemicolectomy are

1. The patient is placed in a head-down position, with transverse mesocolon stretched out, as described above.

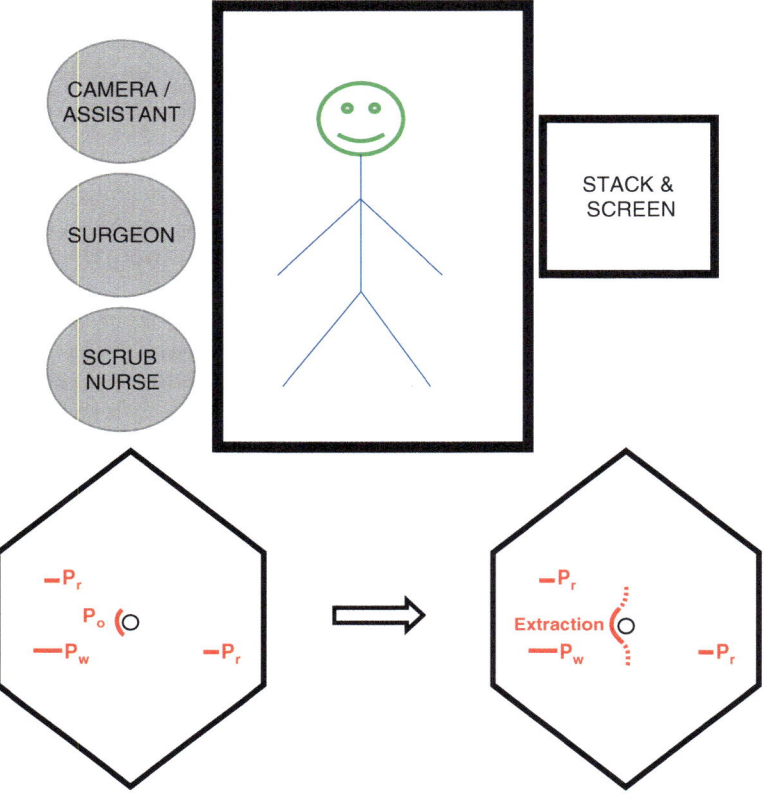

Fig. 3.3 The theatre setup for Lap Left Hemi/Sigmoid Colectomy/Proctectomy. P_o—12 mm Optical Port, P_w—12 mm Working instrument port, P_r—5 mm Retracting instrument port

2. The visceral peritoneum is incised in the sulcus left lateral to the tented middle colic pedicle, above the "horizon" of the pancreas, and the lesser sac is entered by careful dissection through the mesocolon. The posterior stomach should become apparent at this point. The mesocolon can then safely be divided lateral to the middle colics to the tail of the pancreas.
3. The left mesocolon is stretched antero-laterally and incised superior to the inferior mesenteric vein as it courses towards the inferior pancreas, adjacent to the duodeno-jejunal flexure. The mesocolon can then be divided to meet the previous dissection so the medial aspect of the splenic flexure is fully mobilized.
4. The mesocolic dissection can then be taken in the inferior direction towards the pelvis. It may be easy to identify the left colic vessels in thin patients and divide these at the root of the mesocolon, sparing the main trunk of the IMA and IMV. If not readily evident, the IMV can be divided at the root of the mesentery. The left colic artery comes off the IMA and usually travels near IMV towards the angle

of the splenic flexure, so it can be divided at the same level. For true proximal left colon tumors, the author tries to preserve the sigmoid and haemorrhoidal branches of the IMA so that the sigmoid distal to the anastomosis is well vascularised.
5. Attention should then be turned to taking the distal transverse colon off the greater omentum and mobilizing the splenic flexure, as above. The lateral parieto-colic ligament should be divided along the white line of Toldt to the pelvic brim, ensuring that the entire left colon is mobile, to the proximal sigmoid. It may also be necessary to take the sigmoid off the parietes to avoid any tension in the bowel.
6. There should be at least 10 cm of mobilized colon distal and proximal to the tumor, with the nearest lymph node basin excised, down to the root of the mesocolon. Extraction, as described above. For a true left colon tumor, it is likely to be difficult to insert a circular stapler trans-anally, up to the distal end of the mobilized bowel, for an end-to-end anastomosis, and the author's preference is a sutured end—end anastomosis. The operation concluded as described above.

Sigmoid Colectomy

The MDT process must be robust to ascertain that the lesion is not an upper rectal lesion, and is appropriate to be managed with the requisite segmental colonic resection [18, 19]. Rectal neoplasms with mesorectal envelopes must be understood to be a separate entity. Patients with rectal lesions require different staging and treatment algorithms (see Chap. 5). The general convention is that lesions within 15 cm of the anorectal angle are in the "surgical" rectum. At laparoscopy, the rectum commences where two of the sigmoid taenia coli fuse to become the single broad anterior rectal longitudinal muscle. It is generally advised that the term "recto-sigmoid" cancer is avoided, and a tumor is defined as clearly sigmoid, or rectal, in location.

The patient is placed in a low Lloyd-Davis position, with both arms preferably tucked into the body. If there are no boots, then the legs can be abducted flat and secured on vein boards. Malpositioning of the legs results in complications including peroneal palsy, and compartment syndrome—so the operating surgeon must take full responsibility for this, BEFORE scrubbing up. It is also important to move the legs after 3–4 h of operating if the patient has been in the same position.

Access as described previously. Two working ports are inserted under vision on the right side of the abdomen—the lower port is a 12 mm port to allow insertion of the linear stapler. A further fourth port can be inserted on the left side if further traction or mobilization of the splenic flexure is needed. The initial setup of the patient, and surgical field, for sigmoid colectomy is important to get right and is worth taking extra time before commencing any operation, as initiating dissection in the wrong plane or location can easily lead to situations that are difficult to retrieve, with damage to retroperitoneal vessels, nerves and structures.

The essential steps of laparoscopic sigmoid colectomy are

1. The patient is placed in head head-down position with transverses colon above the liver. The small bowel is retracted cephalad and to the right side, before a lateral tilt, with the left side upwards. For a patient with a floppy sigmoid loop, the sigmoid loop should be delivered out of the pelvis so that the mesosigmoid and upper mesorectum are in a straight line, under some tension. In this position, the aorta is evident posteriorly and is the "horizon" for the medial to lateral dissection. The gentle arc of the superior haemorrhoidal artery can be identified, coursing into the pelvis. This is an important landmark to define, following this arc cephalad leads to the IMA pedicle as it comes off the aorta, and following this arc caudal leads into the correct plane for a total mesorectal excision.
2. The IMA pedicle is identified by tracing the SHA arc. The visceral peritoneum is incised in the sulcus just posterior to the tented pedicle, and the embryological plane between the mesocolon and retroperitoneum is entered. Careful blunt dissection in this plane should lead to the retroperitoneal structures "dropping" from the back of the mesosigmoid, in particular the ureter which is always medial to the gonadal vessels. As a rule, if the iliac vessels or psoas muscle are evident, the dissection is too posterior.
3. This mainly avascular plane can then be developed, usually by blunt dissection laterally, to the posterior aspect of the white line of Toldt. Once the ureter and gonadal vessels are identified, the IMA pedicle can be gradually thinned out, and divided. The hypogastric nerves should be identified and spared. As a rough rule of thumb, especially in obese patients, this author aims to take the IMA around 7/8 mm above the aorta if the nerves are not readily identifiable, dissecting tightly on the posterior aspect of the IMA/SHA (Fig. 3.4).
4. The retro-colic cave is developed supero-medially lifting the mesocolon off Gerota's peri-nephric fascia. The IMV can be identified, dissected, and divided

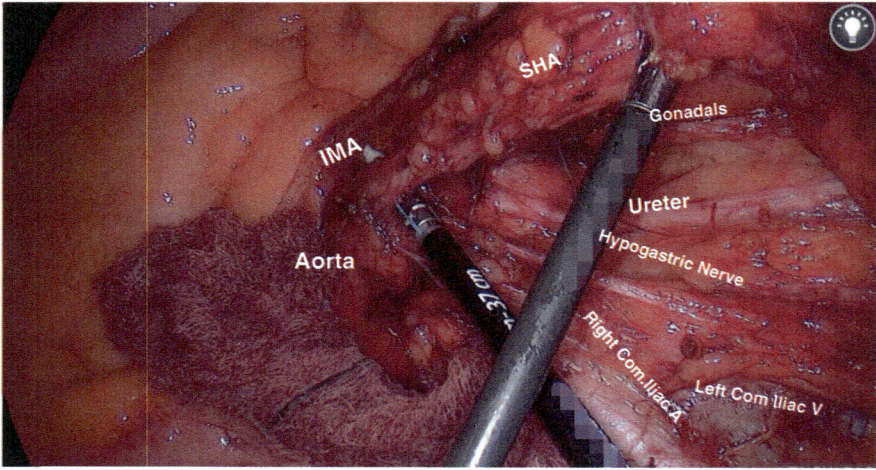

Fig. 3.4 Dissection of the IMA just before division, with major retro-peritoneal structures identified before division of IMA

where it courses more superiorly in the mesocolon. The IMV is like a bowstring within the left mesocolon, tethering the left colon to the retroperitoneum at the level of the tail of the pancreas. Its division is necessary so that the mobilized colon can reach the pelvis without tension for creating anastomoses.
5. The splenic flexure does not always need to be mobilized for a tension-free anastomosis, but if required, the IMV is divided close to the mesocolic root, the dissection developed cephalad, taking care to dissect anterior to the pancreatic tail, then into the lesser sac posterior to the distal transverse colon. The splenic flexure can be taken down off the omentum, spleen, and parietes as described above.
6. The distal resection margin depends on the exact location of the tumor, aiming for a distal resection margin of at least 5 cm. The upper mesorectum can be thinned down to the rectal muscle tube. It is the author's practice to infuse ICG at this point, to confirm good blood supply at this level of the rectum, which is then divided with a linear stapler. A grasper is secured close to the colonic staple line and locked, then extraction of the bowel as described above.
7. The mesocolon proximal to the tumor is divided down to the bowel at the proposed proximal resection margin, and ICG is used to confirm the bowel is well-perfused at this point (Fig. 3.5). The bowel is divided with a blade, then the end closed over the anvil of a circular stapler with a purse-string suture and returned to the abdomen.
8. The bowel is returned to the abdomen, and the pneumo-peritoneum re-established. The circular stapler is introduced through the anus and carefully guided up to the rectal staple line. The proximal colon is delivered adjacent to this. There should be no tension on the proximal colon, if there is any tension, this needs to be addressed at this point. The spike of the stapler is brought through the staple line preferably centrally, and docked with the anvil spike securely, and bowel ends brought together. It is the author's practice to infuse ICG at this point and also to confirm both sides of the anastomosis are well perfused—this is the most important use of ICG, and if only going to be used once per case, this is the most crucial step, before forming the anastomosis.
9. Many authorities now recommend a triple check to minimize the dreaded complication of anastomotic leak: ICG fluorescence angiography PLUS an air leak test to check the anastomosis remains airtight when distended PLUS flexible sigmoidoscopic assessment of the luminal aspect to ensure no obvious defects, with the mucosa pink and healthy on both sides of the staple line.

Post-operative Complications

It is now well-established that a crucial concept in post-operative care is "rescuing" patients with complications. There is a statistical inevitability about surgical complications, even in the very best hands, however, "failure to rescue" is what separates even good surgical systems, from truly excellent ones. Foundational to managing complications well are humility, and vigilance, for early symptoms or

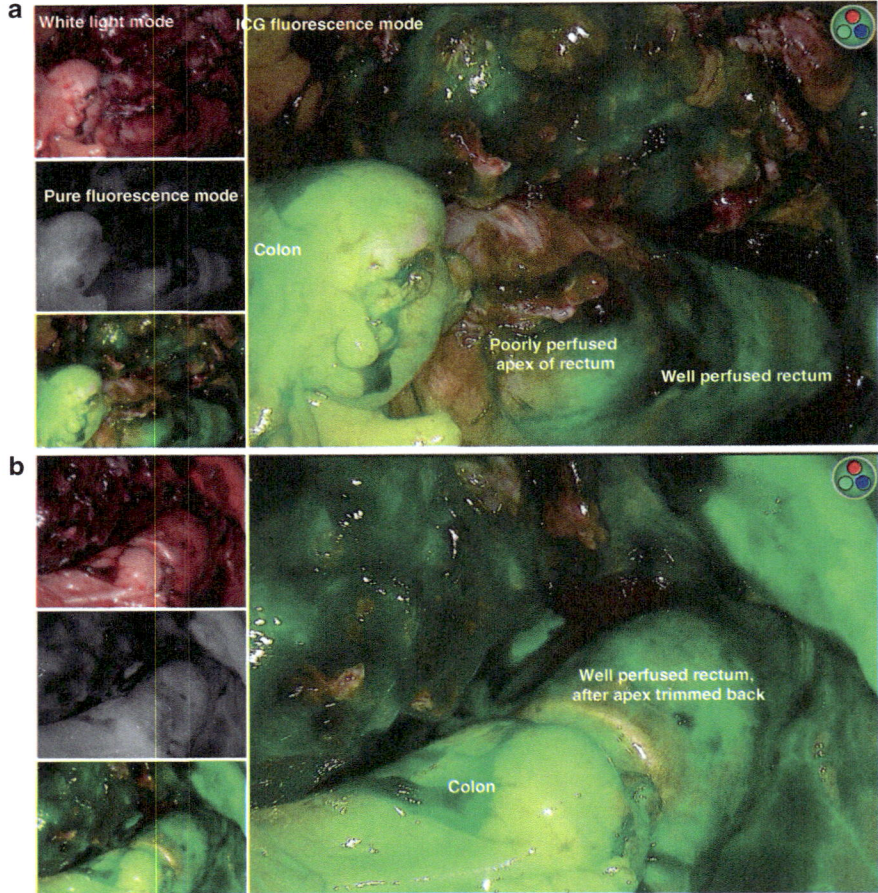

Fig. 3.5 ICG infused after sigmoid colectomy at the formation of stapled colorectal anastomosis: poor perfusion demonstrated in rectal apex (**a**) so trimmed back to healthy, well-vascularised rectum before formation of anastomosis (**b**)

signs of complication. In a resource-limited setting, this may be less dependent on daily, sequential lab tests, and cross-sectional imaging, though where available, these adjuncts are invaluable to supplement, but must never replace clinical assessment. One of the benefits of laparoscopic surgery is that there is also the opportunity for diagnostic re-laparoscopy in managing post-op patients.

Special Notes

Technological advances continue apace. The next surgical revolution is the robotic one, with the multi-dimensional instrument dexterity and optical stability of the robotic platform widely perceived as a game-changer. Added to this is the intangible but no less valuable reality that the surgeon can now perform surgery sitting comfortably at a console, without the occupational postural musculoskeletal problems from long surgical procedures.

Other laparoscopic techniques—single incision laparoscopic surgery, complete mesocolic excision—have their advocates. However, the scientific data is equivocal, and the vast majority of laparoscopic colorectal surgery generally follow the multiport, stepwise approach, laid out above, with clear variations according to surgical experience, practice, and patient factors.

References

1. Jacobs M, Verdaja JC, Goldstein H. Minimally invasive colon resection (laparoscopic colectomy). Surg Laparosc Endosc. 1991;1:144–50.
2. Fowler DL, White SA. Laparoscopy-assisted sigmoid resection. Surg Laparosc Endosc. 1991;1:183–8.
3. The Clinical Outcomes of Surgical Therapy Study Group. A comparison of laparoscopically assisted and open colectomy for colon cancer. N Engl J Med. 2004;350 2050–9.
4. Guillou PJ, Quirke P, Thorpe H, et al. Short-term endpoints of conventional versus laparoscopic-assisted surgery in patients with colorectal cancer (MRC CLASICC trial): multicentre, randomised controlled trial. Lancet. 2005;365:1718–26.
5. Veldkamp R, Kuhry E, Hop WCJ, et al. Laparoscopic surgery versus open surgery for colon cancer: short-term outcomes of a randomised trial. Lancet Oncol. 2005;7:477–84.
6. The Colon Cancer Laparoscopic or Open Resection Group. Survival after laparoscopic surgery versus open surgery for colon cancer: long-term outcome of a randomised clinical trial. Lancet. 2008;10:44–52. https://doi.org/10.1016/S1470-2045(08)70310-3.
7. Law WL, Lee YM, Choi HK, et al. Impact of laparoscopic resection for colorectal cancer on operative outcomes and survival. Ann Surg. 2003;245:1–7.
8. Wu Q, Wei M, Ye Z, et al. Laparoscopic colectomy versus open colectomy for treatment of transverse colon cancer: a systematic review and meta-analysis. J Laparoendosc Adv Surg Tech A. 2017;27:1038–50.
9. Mike M, Kano N. Reappraisal of the vascular anatomy of the colon and consequences for the definition of surgical resection. Dig Surg. 2013;30:383–92.
10. Ziabari Y, Wigmore T, Kasivisvanathan R. The multidisciplinary team approach for high-risk and major cancer surgery. BJA Educ. 2017;17:255–61.
11. Dunin De Skrzynno SCJ, Di Maggio F. Surgical consent in sub-Saharan Africa: a modern challenge for the humanitarian surgeon. Trop Doc. 2018;48:217–20.
12. Ogundiran TO, Adebamowo CA. Surgeons' opinions and practice of informed consent in Nigeria. J Med Ethics. 2010;36:741–5.
13. Green B, Oeppen RS, Smith DW, Brennan PA. Challenging hierarchy in healthcare teams—ways to flatten gradients to improve teamwork and patient care. Br J Oral Maxillofac Surg. 2017;55:449–53.

14. Gustafsson UO, Scott MJ, Hubner M, et al. Guidelines for perioperative care in elective colorectal surgery: enhanced recovery after surgery (ERAS®) society recommendations: 2018. World J Surg. 2019;43:659–95.
15. www.erassociety.org
16. Hasson HM. A modified instrument and method for laparoscopy. Am J Obstet Gynaecol. 1971;110:886–7.
17. Milone M, Manigrasso M, Elmore U, et al. Short- and long-term outcomes after transverse colectomy versus extended colectomy for transverse colon cancer. A systematic review and meta-analysis. Int J Color Dis. 2019;34:201–7.
18. Loffeld RJLF, Flens M, Fransen G, den Boer FC, van Bochove A. The localisation of cancer in the sigmoid, rectum, or rectosigmoid junction using endoscopy or radiology—what is the most accurate method? J Gastrointest Oncol. 2014;5:469–73.
19. D'Souza N, de Neree Tot Babberich MPM, Lord A, et al. The rectosigmoid problem. Surg Oncol. 2018;27:521–5.

Chapter 4
Robot-Assisted Laparoscopic Colorectal Surgery

Emeka Ray-Offor and Olusegun Komolafe

Introduction

Since the introduction of laparoscopic colorectal surgery in 1992, well-established advantages in abdominal surgery such as early recovery, minimized morbidity, and scarring and other aesthetic advantages have been documented [1]. However, there are limitations to conventional laparoscopic surgery. These include the two-dimensional (2D) image which requires the surgeon to sometimes adopt an uncomfortable position to obtain the best working angle and simultaneously the best view [2]. A limited 4-degree freedom range of movement from conventional rigid laparoscopic instruments in addition to fatigue-induced tremors can reduce precision with adverse effects. The fulcrum effect at the incision site on the anterior abdominal necessitates a counterintuitive downward arm movement on an instrument handle to perform an upward movement at the tip and vice versa [3]. In rectal surgeries, technical problems arising from the location of the tumor, working space challenges from limited pelvic space, and tumor size also are encountered [4, 5]. To overcome some of these limitations of conventional laparoscopic surgery, robotic surgical systems (RSSs) were introduced.

The use of an automatic machine (robot) able to take some tasks from human hands was first applied to surgery in 1985 for image-guided biopsy in neurosurgery

E. Ray-Offor (✉)
College of Health Sciences, University of Port Harcourt, Choba, Rivers State, Nigeria

Colorectal/Minimal Access Surgery Unit, Department of Surgery, University of Port Harcourt Teaching Hospital, Port Harcourt, Rivers State, Nigeria
e-mail: emeka.ray-offor@uniport.edu.ng

O. Komolafe
University Hospital Wishaw, Wishaw, Scotland

University of Glasgow, Glasgow, Scotland

[6]. The application of this innovative technique was soon extended to urology then orthopaedics with robot-assisted colorectal surgery first introduced in 2002 [7]. RSSs are increasingly used with about 200,000 operations performed worldwide annually [8]. One of the most promising inventions in abdominal robotic surgery is the DaVinci® system (Intuitive Surgical, Sunnyvale, CA, USA) launched in 2000 with newer models later developed [9]. This RSS comprises a remote immersive ergonomic surgeon console with a binocular three-dimensional (3D) vision of a surgical field connected by cables to a surgical cart with arms docked on the patient for real-time manipulation of the camera and the surgical instruments. Also, an equipment cart holds the monitors, light source, energy devices, etc. The advanced features provided by RSSs over conventional laparoscopy include 3D vision, on a stable platform, tremor or motion scaling of instruments within the surgical field, wristed instruments having 7-degrees of freedom, and improved ergonomics for the operating surgeon.

A review of the literature collectively concludes that robotic surgery is safe and efficacious, with equivalent oncological outcomes and complication rates; although operative times are significantly longer, the length of hospital stay has been reported to be shorter with lower conversion rates to open surgery during pelvic surgery [10, 11]. Despite the value added to surgical care by RSSs, there are limitations to the wide-scale adoption of robotic laparoscopic surgery with the lead being cost-related. Robotic surgery is an expensive health care provision that costs about USD 2 to 3 million for the capital acquisition, limited-use instruments, surgical team training, maintenance, and repair in addition to costs from the increased OR time. A retrospective analysis from the National Inpatient Sample database revealed additional healthcare average costs of about USD 2000 for robot-assisted laparoscopic surgeries compared to conventional laparoscopic surgery [$12,340 ± $5880 vs $10,227 ± $4986 ($p < 0.001$), respectively] [12]. Hence surgical volume is crucial in building a business case for RSS for hospital management. Many colorectal procedures such as sigmoid and low anterior resections require multiple quadrant steps creating the need for redocking of the system. The newer model da Vinci Xi® launched in 2014 addresses the shortcomings of the earlier introduced da Vinci Si® system with operating arms that rotate as a group connected to an overhead boom enabling the ability to perform multi-quadrant surgery through a single docking (Fig. 4.1) [13]. Other drawbacks to robotic surgery include the bulkiness of the robotic equipment, lack of tactile and force feedback to the surgeon, and risk of mechanical failure.

Fig. 4.1 da Vinci xi Robotic Surgery system

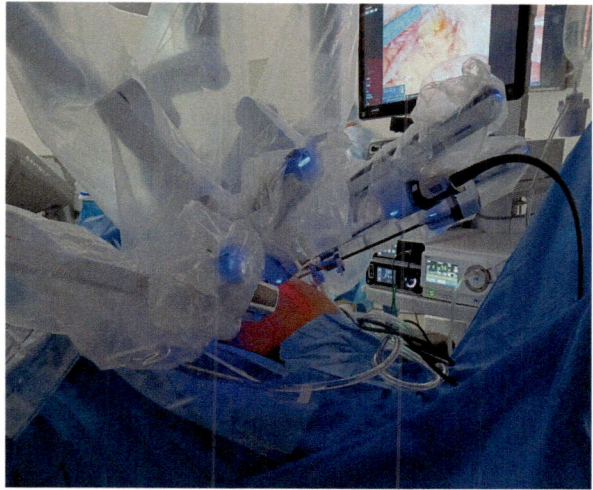

Indications in Colorectal Surgery

The indications for robotic surgery are much the same as those for laparoscopic surgery. In colorectal surgery, the three main colorectal operations where robotic surgery has found the most use are rectal cancer surgery, right hemicolectomy, and ventral mesh rectopexy [14].

Rectal Cancer Surgery

RSSs facilitate technically challenging total mesorectal excision with intracorporeal anastomoses, vascular dissection, and lymphadenectomy in complex anatomical spaces in the pelvis near nerves and vascular structures. The types of resections include anterior resection, low anterior resection, ultra-low anterior resection, abdominoperineal resection, and Hartmann resection. Sphincter-preserving surgeries can be performed with better precision with less conversion to open surgery [15]. These include intersphincteric resection, partial Denonvilliers' fascia excision for anteriorly located rectal cancer, especially in the setting of neoadjuvant chemoradiotherapy and the partial excision of the levator ani muscle for low-lying rectal cancer invading the ipsilateral levator ani muscle.

Right Hemicolectomy

Robotic right hemicolectomy has the advantage of easier facilitation of intracorporeal anastomosis [14]. Ileocolic anastomosis in standard laparoscopy is commonly performed extracorporeally, with the bowel exteriorized through a mini-laparotomy leading to the potential risk of incisional hernia. When the ileocolic anastomosis is performed intracorporeally as facilitated by RSS, the need to mobilize the transverse colon fully is obviated and the extraction site can be smaller. This cumulatively can lead to an earlier return to bowel function, in addition to reduced surgical site infection and incisional hernia rates. Complete mesocolic excision, as facilitated by robotic surgery, with central vascular ligation for right-sided colon cancer, is suggested to offer superior oncological outcomes and a possible survival advantage when compared with standard D2 lymphadenectomy [16].

Ventral Mesh Rectopexy

Pelvic floor reconstructive surgery is an emerging field of application for robotic platforms. The clarity of vision in narrow anatomical areas, facilitated dissection and intracorporeal suturing in ventral rectopexy are often indicated as prime reasons why surgeons choose a robotic approach to perform abdominal pelvic organ prolapse reconstructive procedures (Fig. 4.2a–c). An international panel of experts recommends robotic surgery over standard laparoscopy especially for obese patients and for patients with previous abdominal surgeries and complex cases of advanced or multicompartmental prolapse, relapsed/recurrent prolapse, or previous reconstructive surgery with meshes [17].

Contraindications

The contraindications to robotic surgery are like laparoscopy and include hemodynamic instability and cardiorespiratory compromise. Patients with local invasion of adjacent structures, bowel obstruction, perforation of the colon, and/or significant hemorrhage are typically treated with open surgery. The relative contraindications include emergency surgery and previous abdominal surgery with extensive adhesions.

Fig. 4.2 (**a–c**) Robotic ventral mesh rectopexy. (**a**) Peritoneal dissection. (**b**) Mesh placement. (**c**) Suture fixation of mesh

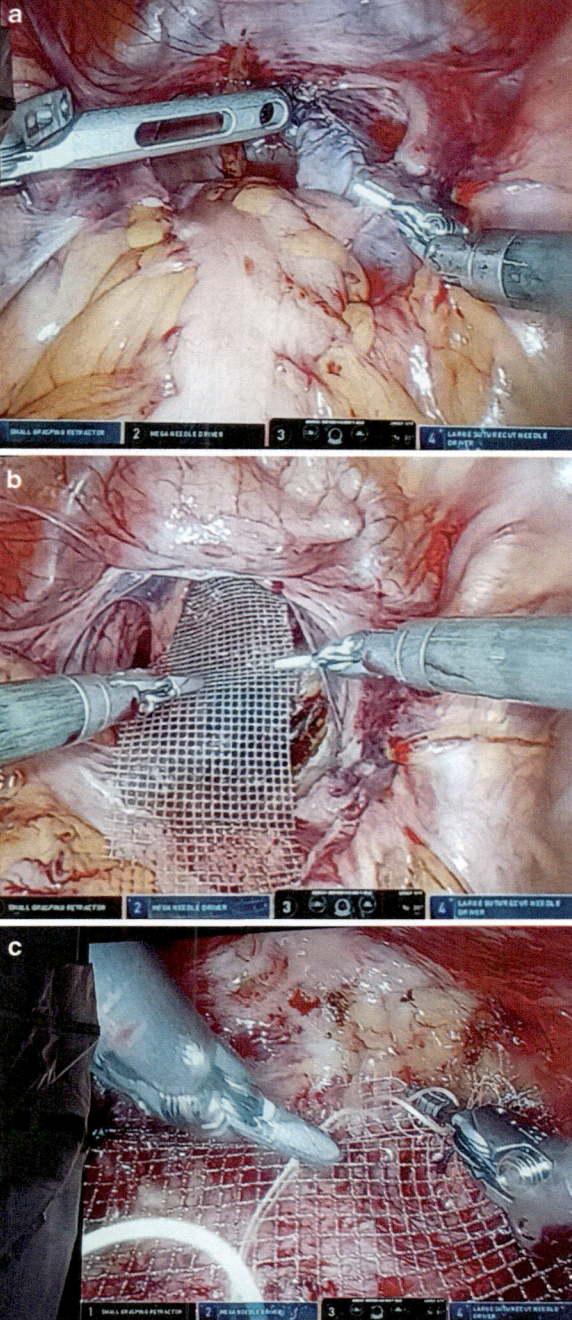

Port Placement

A sound understanding of proper port placement in robotic surgery is essential. Port placement is dependent on the quadrant(s) of the abdomen where the surgery is being performed, technique (hybrid, single-, double- or triple-docking) and surgeons' preference [18]. The port placement for robotic left hemicolectomy or total mesorectal excision is herein described. Typically, open access is used to carefully place a periumbilical 12 mm optical trocar (da Vinci Xi telescope is 8.5 mm). For the robotic working arms, da Vinci 8-mm reusable cannulas with disposable seals are carefully placed under direct vision on either side of the optical trocar at least 8 cm from the umbilicus along the mid-clavicular line to achieve triangulation of instruments and avoid collision of robotic arms (Fig. 4.3). An additional 8 mm working port is sited at the Palmers point under direct vision at a similar distance superiorly. An assistant port is created in the subcostal area of the right upper abdomen along the anterior axillary line. Retention sutures can be used to secure the ports.

The da Vinci single port (SP) robot is specifically designed for endoluminal surgery with a 25-mm SP robotic trocar that allows for the insertion of the robotic camera and three instruments within a confined space.

A critical part of docking is also positioning of the boom and manipulation of the robotic arms to allow greater patient clearance and optimize instrument reach. This point allows for less robotic arm collision and ease in the progression of the case, eventually resulting in decreased operative time. For left colon and TME surgery, the docking is on the left side of the patient on the operating table with precaution exercised to ensure that the patient's knees are low-lying, to prevent collisions with the robotic arms (Fig. 4.4). The contrary is the case for right hemicolectomy. Once docked and robotic arms connected to ports, the table should not be unduly adjusted unless ports are first disengaged.

A new modular RSS, the Versius surgical robotic system, offers several benefits such as articulated instruments that pass through conventional 5 mm ports, compact

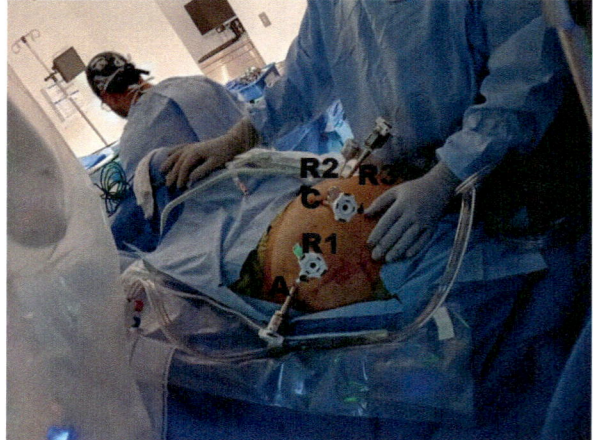

Fig. 4.3 Port placement for splenic flexure and left colon mobilization (R1-arm for monopolar scissors or cautery hook; R2-arm 2 for Maryland or fenestrated bipolar forceps; R3-arm for tip-up fenestrated grasper, A-assistant port, C-camera port)

Fig. 4.4 Robotic arms docked on the right side of the patient's abdomen

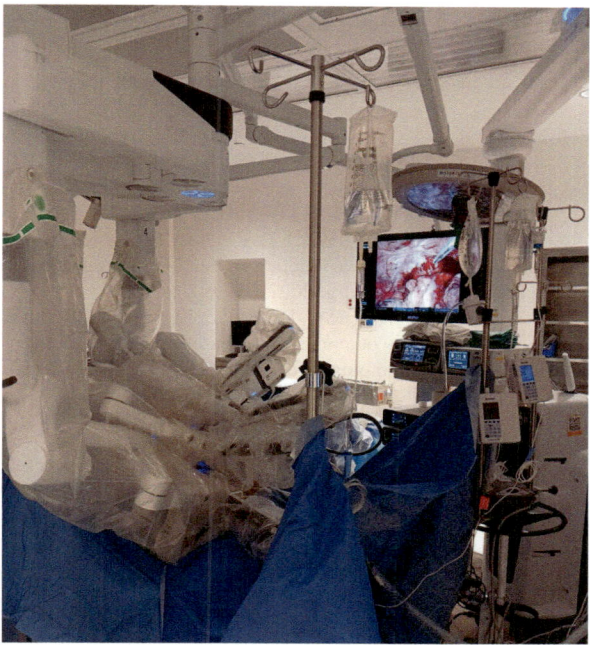

arms for easier maneuverability and patient access, the ability to mimic conventional port placements, and adaptive machine learning concepts [19, 20].

Training in Robotic Colorectal Surgery

The interest and enthusiasm for robot-assisted laparoscopic surgery has remarkably increased, but every new technology requires training. A meta-analysis of studies using a CUSUM sequential analysis in phases of robotic practice calculated the mean number of cases required for the surgeon to be classed as an expert in robotic surgery for rectal cancer to be 39 patients [21]. The need for additional surgical training for the surgical team is pertinent. Many curricula are available with didactic courses comprising patient-side and console training, but their contents are inconsistent; the availability and nature of hands-on training offered by these curriculums are widely variable [22]. In the United States, the Society of American Gastrointestinal and Endoscopic Surgeon Robotic Masters Series, Fundamental Skills of Robot-Assisted Surgery training program, and the Robotics Training Network curriculum have on-site training facilitating expert feedback on surgical techniques and robot maintenance [23]. Advancements in virtual reality simulators have facilitated their integration into robotic-assisted surgery training. Intuitive Surgical offers the software of a robotic trainer mounted on the robotic console with several abstract drills and scoring systems that teach basic instrument and camera manipulation.

References

1. Jacobs M, Verdeja JC, Goldstein HS. Minimally invasive colon resection (laparoscopic colectomy). Surg Laparosc Endosc. 1991;1(3):144–50.
2. Morris B. Robotic surgery: applications, limitations, and impact on surgical education. MedGenMed. 2005;7(3):72.
3. Oppenheimer P, Weghorst S, MacFarlane M, Sinanan M. Immersive surgical robotic interfaces. Stud Health Technol Inform. 1999;62:242–8.
4. Noel JK, Fahrbach K, Estok R, Cella C, Frame D, Linz H, Cima RR, Dozois EJ, Senagore AJ. Minimally invasive colorectal resection outcomes: short term comparison with open procedures. J Am Coll Surg. 2007;204:291–307.
5. Targarona EM, Balagué C, Pernas JC, Martinez C, Berindoague R, Gich I, et al. Can we predict an immediate outcome after laparoscopic rectal surgery? Multivariate analysis of clinical, anatomic, and pathologic features after 3-dimensional reconstruction of the pelvic anatomy. Ann Surg. 2008;247:642–9.
6. Kwoh YS, Hou J, Jonckheere EA, Hayati S. A robot with improved absolute positioning accuracy for CT guided stereotactic brain surgery. IEEE Trans Biomed Eng. 1988;35:153–60.
7. Weber PA, Merola S, Wasielewski A, Ballantyne GH. Telerobotic-assisted laparoscopic right and sigmoid colectomies for benign disease. Dis Colon Rectum. 2002;45:1689–94.
8. Gachabayov M, You K, Kim SH, et al. Meta-analysis of the impact of the learning curve in robotic rectal cancer surgery on histopathologic outcomes. Surg Technol Int. 2019;34:139–55.
9. Sung GT, Gill IS. Robotic laparoscopic surgery: a comparison of the DA Vinci and Zeus systems. Urology. 2001;58(6):893–8.
10. Bhama AR, Obias V, Welch KB, et al. A comparison of laparoscopic and robotic colorectal surgery outcomes using the American College of Surgeons National Surgical Quality Improvement Program (ACS NSQIP) database. Surg Endosc. 2016;30(4):1,576–84.
11. Tam MS, Kaoutzanis C, Mullard AJ, et al. A population-based study comparing laparoscopic and robotic outcomes in colorectal surgery. Surg Endosc. 2016;30(2):455–63.
12. Khorgami Z, Li WT, Jackson TN, Howard CA, Sclabas GM. The cost of robotics: an analysis of the added costs of robotic-assisted versus laparoscopic surgery using the National Inpatient Sample. Surg Endosc. 2019;33(7):2217–21.
13. Katsuno H, Hanai T, Masumori K, et al. Robotic surgery for rectal cancer: operative technique and review of the literature. J Anus Rectum Colon. 2020;4(1):14–24.
14. Sivathondan PC, Jayne DG. The role of robotics in colorectal surgery. Ann R Coll Surg Engl. 2018;100(Suppl 7):42–9.
15. Park SY, Choi GS, Park JS, et al. Short-term clinical outcome of robot–assisted intersphincteric resection for low rectal cancer: a retrospective comparison with conventional laparoscopy. Surg Endosc. 2013;27(1):48–55.
16. West NP, Hohenberger W, Weber K, et al. Complete mesocolic excision with central vascular ligation produces an oncologically superior specimen compared with standard surgery for carcinoma of the colon. J Clin Oncol. 2010;28(2):272–8.
17. Simoncini T, Panattoni A, Aktas M, Ampe J, Betschart C, Bloemendaal ALA, et al. Robot-assisted pelvic floor reconstructive surgery: an international Delphi study of expert users. Surg Endosc. 2023;37(7):5215–25.
18. Lee JL, Alsaleem HA, Kim JC. Robotic surgery for colorectal disease: review of current port placement and future perspectives. Ann Surg Treat Res. 2020;98(1):31–43.
19. Haig F, Medeiros ACB, Chitty K, Slack M. Usability assessment of versius, a new robot-assisted surgical device for use in minimal access surgery. BMJ Surg Interv Health Technol. 2020;2:e000028.
20. Morton J, Hardwick RH, Tilney HS, Gudgeon AM, Jah A, Stevens L, et al. Preclinical evaluation of the versius surgical system, a new robot-assisted surgical device for use in minimal access general and colorectal procedures. Surg Endosc. 2021;35:2169–77.

21. Jiménez-Rodríguez RM, Rubio-Dorado-Manzanares M, Díaz-Pavón JM, Reyes-Díaz ML, Vazquez-Monchul JM, Garcia-Cabrera AM, Padillo J, De la Portilla F. Learning curve in robotic rectal cancer surgery: current state of affairs. Int J Color Dis. 2015;31(12):1807–15.
22. Wang RS, Ambani SN. Robotic surgery training: current trends and future directions. Urol Clin North Am. 2021;48:137–46.
23. Chen R, Rodrigues Armijo P, Krause C, SAGES Robotic Task Force, Siu KC, Oleynikov D. A comprehensive review of robotic surgery curriculum and training for residents, fellows, and postgraduate surgical education. Surg Endosc. 2020;34(1):361–7.

Part II
Rectum

Chapter 5
Laparoscopic Anterior Resection

Emeka Ray-Offor, Sameh Hany Emile, and Nir Horesh

Introduction

The mid and late twentieth century witnessed an evolution in surgical practice with a wide application of minimally invasive techniques to surgeries involving the abdomen and pelvis. Minimally invasive procedures comprise surgical techniques with smaller incisions resulting in a shorter wound healing time and decreased postoperative pain and risk of infection. The spectrum of minimally invasive procedures for rectal cancer ranges from advanced trans-anal excision, pure laparoscopic, combined trans-anal, and laparoscopic to robot-assisted techniques. Selection of the appropriate procedure is complex and should ideally involve a multi-disciplinary discussion. A careful individualized weighing of the risks, benefits, and alternatives for all surgical and non-surgical options is required. Importantly, the choice of surgical technique is dependent on the exact location of the lesion taking into

---

E. Ray-Offor (✉)
College of Health Sciences, University of Port Harcourt, Choba, Rivers State, Nigeria

Colorectal/Minimal Access Surgery Unit, Department of Surgery, University of Port Harcourt Teaching Hospital, Port Harcourt, Rivers State, Nigeria
e-mail: emeka.ray-offor@uniport.edu.ng

S. H. Emile
Colorectal Surgery Department, Ellen Leifer Shulman and Steven Shulman Digestive Disease Institute, Cleveland Clinic Florida, Weston, FL, USA

Department of General Surgery, Faculty of Medicine, Mansoura University, Mansoura, Egypt

Schmidt College of Medicine, Florida Atlantic University, Boca Raton, FL, USA

N. Horesh
Colorectal Surgery Department, Ellen Leifer Shulman and Steven Shulman Digestive Disease Institute, Cleveland Clinic Florida, Weston, FL, USA

Faculty of Medicine, Tel Aviv University, Tel Aviv, Israel

© The Author(s), under exclusive license to Springer Nature Switzerland AG 2024
E. Ray-Offor, R. J. Rosenthal (eds.), *Colorectal & Hernia Laparoscopic Surgery*, https://doi.org/10.1007/978-3-031-63490-1_5

cognizance the reaction to pre-operative oncological treatment, the distance from the anal verge and anorectal ring, orientation within the rectal lumen, and circumferential radial margin [1].

The earliest series of laparoscopic colorectal surgery was reported by Jacobs et al. in 1991 [2]. Slow adoption of laparoscopic colorectal surgery started with initial concerns related to resection margins, possible port site metastases, and tumor cell dissemination during laparoscopic manipulation of the bowel in malignancies of the colon and rectum. [3, 4] Rectal cancer surgeries are technically demanding with the need for total mesorectal excision (TME) and preservation of autonomic nerves for oncological and functional safety. To date, high-level evidence from randomized trials and meta-analyses demonstrate that in selected patients with rectal cancer treated by skilled surgeons, laparoscopic surgery has similar safety, resection margins, and completeness of resection in comparison to open surgery [5–7]. Also, the surgical approach does not appear to influence the likelihood or severity of changes to bowel function known as low anterior resection syndrome (LARS) [8].

Sphincter preservation is a desired goal in rectal surgery when achievable. The advent of new surgical staplers has enabled the safe performance of anastomosis at a very low level [9]. Anterior resection is a sphincter-preserving surgery commonly used to extirpate rectal cancer and it involves resection of the rectum with a primary anastomosis. The procedure is classified as standard, low, or ultra-low based on the extent of dissection and level of anastomosis. A low anterior resection (LAR) is performed within 10 cm from the anal verge (mid and low rectal cancers) in contradistinction to standard anterior resection for which dissection does not extend beyond the peritoneal reflection. An ultra-low resection involves an anastomosis within 2 cm of the anorectal junction. The optimal technique of low anterior resection comprises selective splenic flexure mobilization, high ligation of inferior mesenteric vessels, and intraoperative assessment of anastomotic integrity [10]. A tailored recommendation for stoma creation following low/ultra-low anterior resection for rectal cancer favors laparoscopic ileostomy over laparoscopic colostomy [11].

Relevant Anatomy

The sigmoid colon transitions into the rectum at the cessation of the surgical mesocolon marked by a convergence of the tenia coli and the absence of appendices epiploicae. It is the most distal part of the large intestine commencing opposite the sacral promontory and following the curve of the sacrum to end at the anorectal ring at the level of S3 [12]. The rectum has a variable length of approximately 15 cm from the anal verge. Surgically, the rectum is divided into three parts: low rectum ($\leq$6 cm from the anal verge); mid rectum (from 7 to 11 cm); and upper rectum (from 12 to 15 cm).

The peritoneal covering extends around the front and sides of the upper part of the rectum. The peritoneum is reflected anteriorly in front of the mid-rectum onto the bladder in the male and the posterior vaginal fornix in the female. The rectum is surrounded by a mesorectal fascia, the mesorectum, which consists of connective tissue and fat. The mesorectum is bulkier posteriorly and contains the descending branches of the superior rectal artery, corresponding venous tributaries, and draining lymphatics and nodes. Laterally, it thins out and is closely related to the inferior hypogastric plexus supplied by parasympathetic innervation from nervi erigentes and sympathetic from the superior hypogastric nerves. An avascular areolar tissue plane lies between the mesorectal fascia and the parietal pelvic fascia. This is the ideal plane for dissection as troublesome bleeding may result when the pelvic sacral fascia is breached.

Endoscopically, the rectum is accessible using rigid proctosigmoidoscopy or flexible endoscopy. Three distinct semicircular, inner folds called valves of Houston are noted within the rectum (Fig. 5.1). The superior and inferior rectal valves are located on the left side of the rectum and the more prominent middle rectal valve on the right; however, this is not a constant finding [13]. The anal canal forms proximally where the rectum passes through the pelvic hiatus and joins with the puborectalis muscle, ending distally at the anal verge. It measures about 4 cm in length. At endoscopy, the proximal anal canal has a pink appearance in contrast to the more

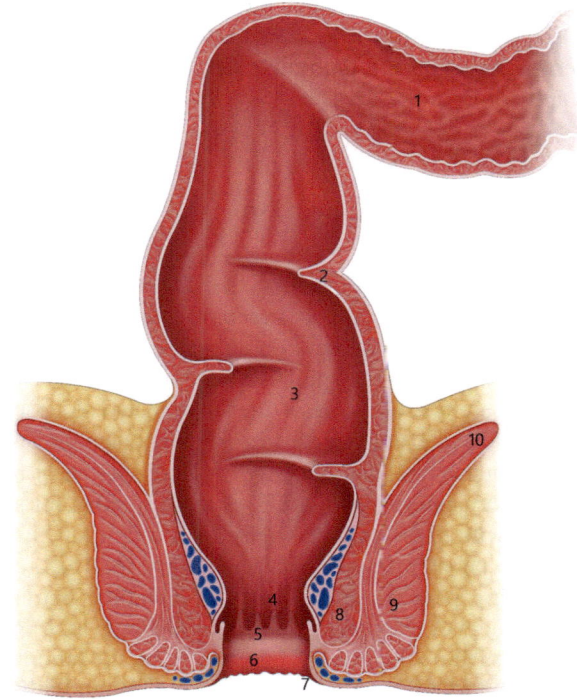

Fig. 5.1 Anatomy of the rectum: (1) Sigmoid colon; (2) Valve of Houston; (3) Rectum; (4) Anal column; (5) Dentate line; (6) Anus; (7) Anal verge; (8) Internal anal sphincter; (9) External anal sphincter; (10) Levator ani muscle (Adapted from Anatomy of the rectum and anus www.shutterstock.com)

reddish rectal mucosa. It is lined by the columnar epithelium of the rectal mucosa. About half to one centimeter proximal to the dentate line, the anal transition zone (ATZ) begins which appears purple and represents an area of gradual transition to squamous epithelium. In this area, the redundant columns of Morgagni are noted with anal crypts at their base, and this forms the rippled dentate line (or pectinate line) The dentate line represents a true division between embryonic endoderm and ectoderm. Distal to the dentate line, is the anoderm that is lined by squamous epithelium and extends for approximately 1.5 cm devoid of hair, sebaceous glands, and sweat glands but becomes thickened, pigmented, and contains hair follicles at the anal verge.

Indications and Contraindications

Primarily, anterior resection is indicated as the surgical treatment for rectosigmoid and rectal cancer located between 1 and 2 cm proximal to the sphincter complex (5–6 cm from the anal verge) and the rectosigmoid junction including secondary tumors by direct invasion e.g., presacral tumors. Non-malignant indications of anterior resection include complex perirectal fistulae, severe pelvic endometriosis, rectal trauma, and large rectal polyps not amenable to endoscopic resection techniques.

Patients who are medically unfit and have severe comorbidities may not be suitable for prolonged surgery in the Trendelenburg position such as anterior resection. Also, patients with poor anal function should be considered for resection with a permanent ostomy, to minimize risk for incontinence after surgery and for a better quality of life.

Preoperative Preparation

Careful patient selection is needed to exclude cases with tumor invasion where oncological safe distal and circumferential resection margins cannot be achieved. Good preoperative preparation comprises a detailed history, physical examination with digital rectal examination, and relevant investigations. The investigations include carcinoembryonic antigen, complete colonoscopy, with chest, and abdominal CT scan to exclude metastases. Pelvic magnetic resonance imaging (MRI) is the gold standard imaging modality for local staging of rectal cancer. The use of transrectal ultrasonography (TRUS) is more suitable for small tumors (T1–2). Primary staging with MRI assists with the detection of locally advanced rectal cancers suitable for neoadjuvant chemoradiotherapy (CRT), guiding surgical planning and identifying poor prognostic factors including extramural vascular invasion and involvement of mesorectal fascia. Re-staging with MRI following neoadjuvant CRT can assess tumor response, complementing the luminal assessment by digital rectal examination and endoscopy, and identify patients with complete pathologic response suitable for a nonsurgical (watch and wait) treatment approach. Positron emission tomography (PET) scan, where available, is a useful adjunct investigation to detect metastases. Ideally, each rectal cancer case is discussed in a multidisciplinary team meeting before surgery. Upon obtaining informed consent, a visit to the stoma nurse is required to mark the stoma site and to educate patients on stoma care and its complications.

The OR theatre equipment comprising advanced laparoscopy set, and flexible endoscope are pre-checked. Enhanced recovery after surgery (ERAS) is followed comprising preoperative education of the patient, optimization of premorbid conditions and nutritional status, and minimal preoperative fasting. Preoperative mechanical bowel preparation and oral antibiotics (neomycin and metronidazole) with administration of intravenous broad-spectrum antibiotics before induction within an hour of incision are recommended for surgical site infection prevention [14]. Prophylactic measures for deep vein thrombosis with pneumatic compression and low molecular weight heparin from the day of surgery before induction should be taken.

Anesthesia

The procedure is performed under general anesthesia with endotracheal intubation. Additionally, a transversus abdominis plane (TAP) block may be performed where this service is available.

Positioning

Great care is taken to carefully pad and protect all areas of potential nerve and body injury. The patient is positioned in modified Lithotomy in stirrups with the buttocks overhanging the operating table by a few centimeters to aid upward and downward manipulation of the intra-anal circular stapler and for good access to the perineum. The arms are tucked to the patient's side for ease of movement of the surgeon and assistants. The patient is securely strapped across the chest onto the operative table. The surgeon is positioned on the right of the patient with the camera operating assistant and an assistant surgeon stands on the opposite side of the patient at the start of surgery.

Technique

Access/Pneumoperitoneum and Trocar Placement

The abdomen, pelvis, perineum, anus, and vagina are prepped and draped in a typical sterile manner. Access to the abdominal cavity can be achieved through several techniques, including the open Hasson technique or the closed Veress needle technique. Some surgeons prefer to gain access guided through an Optiview trocar that allows direct visualization while entering through the different abdominal layers. The latter is often performed in the left upper quadrant to minimize the risk of internal injury. Carbon dioxide pneumoperitoneum of 12–15 mmHg is achieved, then a 30-degree telescope is carefully introduced. In patients with a previous midline lower scar, the primary port is placed in the left upper quadrant with the introduction of the laparoscope to assess adhesions. An infraumbilical port is then created under direct vision and the laparoscope is transferred to this port.

A diagnostic laparoscopy Is performed to evaluate the four quadrants of the abdominal pelvic cavity searching for evidence of peritoneal carcinomatosis, ascites, and liver metastases. The pelvis is assessed for lateral extension of tumor or invasion of adjacent structures to determine the feasibility of sound oncological resection. Two additional ports are carefully placed through horizontal stab wounds under direct vision, one in the right lower quadrant and another in the right upper quadrant.

Medial-to-Lateral Approach

Dissection is commenced at the level of the sacral promontory on the right side of the rectosigmoid colon after tenting the mesentery of the sigmoid colon and retracting anteriorly and laterally. The loose areolar plane between the underside of the sigmoid mesentery and retroperitoneum is identified and the dissection is carefully extended laterally, identifying the gonadal artery, and left stented ureter guided by fluorescence angiography. The ureter is carefully reflected posteriorly out of the dissection path. The incision is extended cephalad to the origin of the IMA which is then skeletonized and ligated proximal to the bifurcation of the left colic artery and inferior rectal artery with a vessel sealing device. The IMV is exposed up to the inferior border of the pancreas near the ligament of Treitz and ligated proximal to any branch point in a similar manner to the IMA. The dissection is continued laterally beneath the sigmoid colon and the left colon mesentery to the left abdominal sidewall exposing the line of Toldt. This avascular tissue is taken down up to the splenic flexure with scissors or an energy device on the displacement of the left/sigmoid colon.

Splenic Flexure Mobilization

The Trendelenburg position is reversed to facilitate this step. A tent is created on the omentum and the lesser sac is entered with an energy device. The omentum is divided preferably using a bipolar energy device to the level of the middle colic vessels. The splenic flexure is mobilized by a combination of dissection towards the distal transverse colon and along the left colon gutter. Selective mobilization of splenic flexure is required for tension-free anastomosis [15].

Lateral-to-Medial Approach

A combination of the right side down and head down tilt of the table is done to displace the small bowel out of the lower abdomen. The initial step involves a gentle medial traction of the sigmoid colon then an incision of the attachment of the visceral and peritoneal peritoneum at the junction of the proximal sigmoid and descending colon at the pelvic brim. The optimal dissection plane is identified and maintained—an avascular areolar tissue anterior to Gerota fascia and retroperitoneal tissue. A combination of blunt and sharp dissection is used to mobilize the left colon along the line of Toldt in a lateral to the medial manner and cephalad direction using monopolar energy or harmonic scalpel while maintaining medial traction. The left colon is mobilized in the same manner up to the splenic flexure. Care should be taken to identify the left stented ureter guided by fluorescence angiography and using the gonadal artery as a landmark in males.

The mesentery is tented by grasping the sigmoid colon and retracting anterior-laterally to identify the IMA. A safe incision is made in the mesentery and extended cephalad to the origin of the IMA which is skeletonized and ligated proximally to the bifurcation of the left colic artery and inferior rectal artery. Ligation is performed with a vessel sealing device (e.g. 10 mm LigaSure Atlas (Covidien), EnSeal (Ethicon), or Hem-o-lok). As previously described for the medial-to-lateral approach, the inferior mesenteric vein (IMV) is exposed up to the inferior border of the pancreas near the ligament of Treitz and ligated proximal to any branch point in a similar manner to IMA. The splenic flexure may then be mobilized as described above.

Pelvic Dissection

Attention is then turned to the pelvis with anterior retraction of the rectosigmoid colon to assist with the identification of the plane between presacral fascia and fascia propria of the rectum posteriorly. Dissection is started and continued in this plane with the right and left hypogastric nerves posteriorly out of harm's way. A total mesorectal mobilization is undertaken dividing Waldeyer's fascia past the tip of the coccyx for a low anterior resection and the lateral stalks. Anteriorly, the plane between the rectum and the seminal vesicles/prostate in males or the vagina in females is carefully dissected. The rectum is circumferentially cleared of fat to facilitate a single firing as multiple firing may increase the risk of anastomotic leak. Under flexible endoscopic guidance, the rectum is then divided with a distal margin of ≥ 2 cm (1–2 cm above the dentate line for ultra-low anterior resection) using a 60-mm endoscopic linear cutting stapler. The pelvis is then filled with water. Again, flexible sigmoidoscopy is performed, and an air-leak test is performed by insufflation of air into the distal stump. Next, the mesentery of the colon is divided with an energy device up to the level of healthy mid-sigmoid colon level.

The entire left colon is exteriorized via an opening created by lengthening the original umbilical incision 4 cm and inserting an Alexis wound protector or by a Pfannenstiel incision and the point of transection is selected. Optionally, the anesthesiologist can administer 3.5 mL of indocyanine green and a 10 mL flush to demonstrate excellent perfusion to 0.2 cm distal to the point selected for the transaction. After transection, a purse string is created with a 2-0 monofilament suture by taking progressive similar-sized seromuscular bites of wall, at the same distance close to the transected margin, around the circumference of the lumen. For efficiency, a purse string clamp is used (Fig. 5.2a). The purse string clamp is applied to the selected point of transection (Fig. 5.2b). Then a Kocher clamp is placed across the specimen end and the bowel is divided between the Kocher clamp and the purse string clamp. A monofilament suture on a Keith needle is then passed back and forth through the purse string clamp. The purse string clamp is then removed. A well-vascularized bowel should bleed from the edge and have healthy pink mucosa. The anvil of a 33-mm circular stapler is easily secured in the lumen (Fig. 5.2c and d) and reintroduced into the abdomen. The Alexis retractor is covered, and the pneumoperitoneum is reestablished. Where a Pfannenstiel incision was used for exteriorization of the transected bowel, this site is then closed and pneumoperitoneum is re-established.

The abdomen and pelvis are again copiously irrigated, and hemostasis secured. The 33 mm circular stapler device is carefully introduced trans-anally until the cartridge rests flush with the distal staple line. The trocar is made to protrude immediately posterior to the midportion of the staple line (Fig. 5.3a). The anvil is replaced over the receptacle trocar (Fig. 5.3b and c). Great care is taken to maintain appropriate anatomic orientation of the colon and its mesentery and exclusion of extraneous structures as the stapler is carefully closed (Fig. 5.3d), and then fired, opened, and gently removed revealing 2 circumferentially full-thickness tissue donuts with a circumferentially intact proximal purse string suture. A repeat of the ICG perfusion assessment is performed (Fig. 5.4a and b).

The four components of the standard technique of quadruple assessment of colorectal and coloanal anastomoses comprise (1) the air leak test; (2) endoscopic visualization; (3) assessment of perfusion with indocyanine green fluorescence angiography (ICGFA); and (4) inspection of both tissue rings ('doughnuts') after creation of a circular stapled anastomosis [16]. The pelvis is filled with water. The

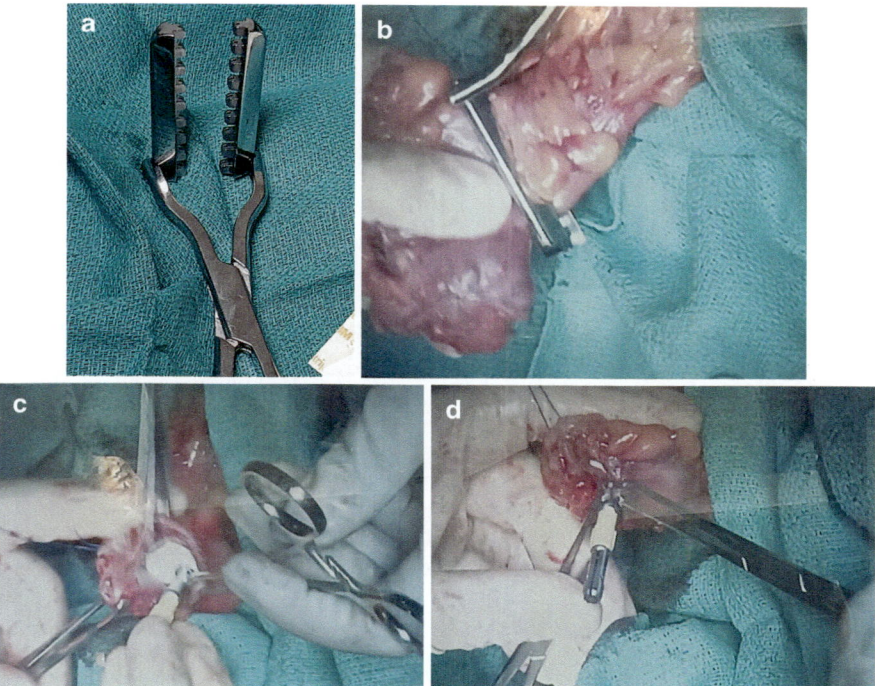

Fig. 5.2 (**a–d**) Extracorporeal preparation of proximal colon for an intracorporeal anastomosis. (**a**) Purse string clamp. (**b**) Purse string clamp applied. (**c**) Insertion of circular stapler anvil. (**d**) Anvil secured with purse string

descending colon is gently occluded, and flexible sigmoidoscopy is performed to show a wide patent, circumferentially intact, airtight, tension-free, hemostatic anastomosis above the dentate line (Fig. 5.5). Any bubbling of fluid on insufflation is assessed and the anastomosis is revised. Additionally, the anaesthesiologist administers an extra 3.5 mL of indocyanine green and 10 mL flush to assess the perfusion of the anastomosis. A pelvic drain (e.g., 19 mm Blake drain) may be placed through a stab wound in the abdominal wall, positioned in the presacral space, and sutured skin with 2-0 Nylon. For patients with a low anastomosis or patients treated with neoadjuvant chemoradiotherapy, a diverting loop ileostomy should be considered as described in Chap. 1 of this book. Fascial layer closure of all port sites >7 mm is done with PDS 1 then subcuticular skin closure of all skin wounds with polyglactin 2.0. Skin dressing is applied. Ureteric stents and orogastric or nasogastric tubes placed intraoperatively are removed at the end of surgery.

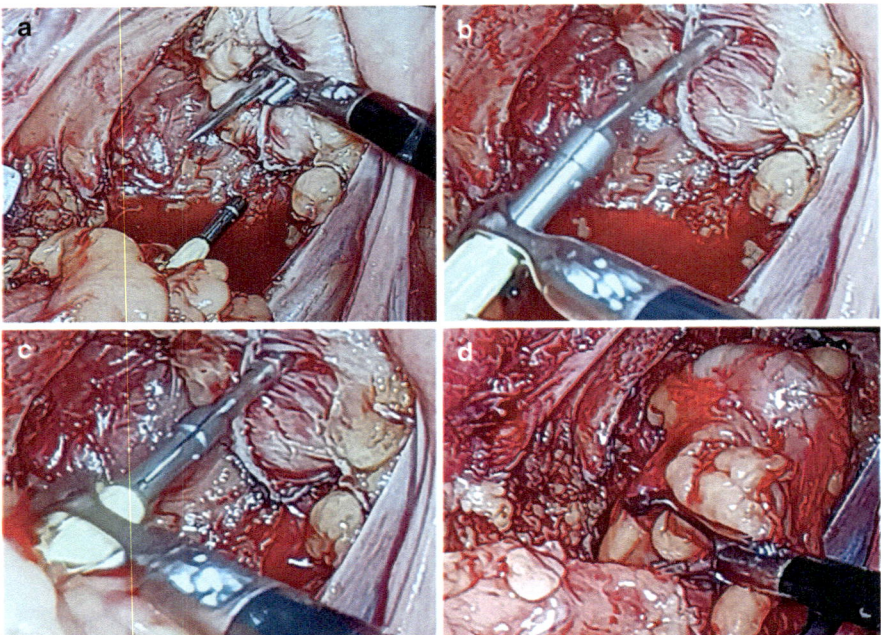

Fig. 5.3 Intracorporeal anastomosis. (**a**) Trocar in the midportion of staple line. (**b**) Aligning trocar and anvil of the circular stapler. (**c**) Aligned anvil and trocar of the circular stapler. (**d**) Orientation of the colon before the firing of the stapler

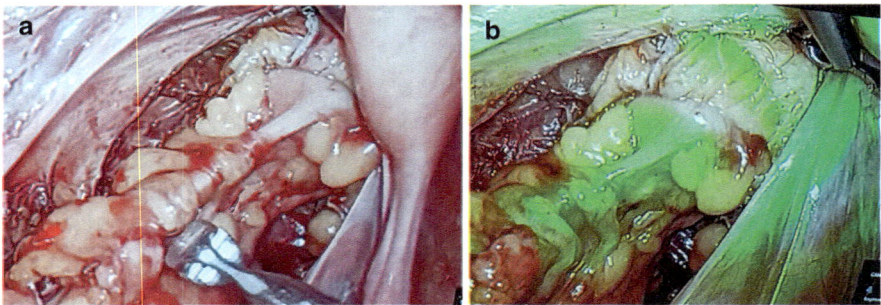

Fig. 5.4 (**a** and **b**) Fluorescence angiography for perfusion assessment

Post-operative Care

Tissue specimens comprising the resected rectosigmoid, and each individually labeled donut are sent to the Pathology laboratory. Prophylaxis for postoperative nausea and vomiting is administered. Adequate analgesia and low molecular weight heparin DVT prophylaxis are maintained. On day 1, oral fluid intake is commenced

5 Laparoscopic Anterior Resection

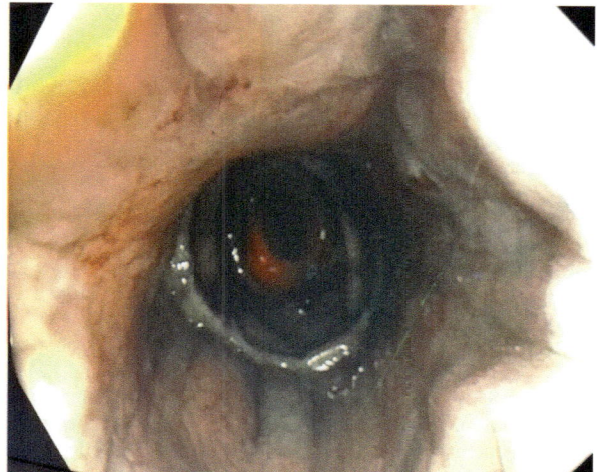

Fig. 5.5 Intraoperative endoscopic assessment of anastomosis

as tolerated, the urethral catheter is removed, and patients are encouraged to ambulate. Respiratory exercises and physical therapy are encouraged to reduce the risk of post-operative complications. The patient is considered for discharge when ambulation, oral nutrition, and intestinal function are established in the absence of complications. Post-operative outpatient clinic visit pathology report is discussed with a follow-up plan instituted according to treatment guidelines based on the pathological outcomes [1].

Special Note

Nearly 75% of the patients who have undergone an anterior resection will be affected by a constellation of bowel dysfunction symptoms including urgency, frequency, fecal incontinence, stool clustering, and incomplete evacuation in the first year following surgery [17]. The complex of symptoms referred to as Low anterior resection syndrome (LARS) can have a significant impact on quality of life (QoL). Notably, the persistence of these symptoms beyond a year of surgery may occur in a quarter of patients who develop LARS [18]. Conservative measures in the management of LARS include changes to diet, anti-diarrhea medications (e.g. loperamide) enemas, and physiotherapy techniques. Transanal irrigation or sacral neuromodulation can be used when conservative measures are not adequate [19].

References

1. Benson AB, Venook AP, Al-Hawary MM, Azad N, Chen Y, Ciombor KK, et al. Rectal cancer, version 2.2022, NCCN clinical practice guidelines in oncology. J Natl Compr Cancer. 2022;20:1139–67.
2. Jacobs M, Verdeja JC, Goldstein HS. Minimally invasive colon resection (laparoscopic colectomy). Surg Laparosc Endosc. 1991;1(3):144–50.
3. Nduka CC, Monson JR, Menzies-Gow N, Darzi A. Abdominal wall metastases following laparoscopy. Br J Surg. 1994;81:648–52.
4. Jayne DG, Thorpe HC, Copeland J, et al. Five-year follow-up of the Medical Research Council CLASICC trial of laparoscopically assisted versus open surgery for colorectal cancer. Br J Surg. 2010;97:1638–45.
5. Clinical Outcomes of Surgical Therapy Study Group. A comparison of laparoscopically assisted and open colectomy for colon cancer. N Engl J Med. 2004;350(20):2050–9.
6. Kang SB, Park JW, Jeong SY, Nam BH, Choi HS, Kim DW, et al. Open versus laparoscopic surgery for mid or low rectal cancer after neoadjuvant chemoradiotherapy (COREAN trial): short-term outcomes of an open-label randomized controlled trial. Lancet Oncol. 2010;11:637–45.
7. van der Pas MH, Haglind E, Cuesta MA, Furst A, Lacy AM, Hop WC, Bonjer HJ, Colorectal cancer Laparoscopic or Open Resection II (COLOR II) Study Group. Laparoscopic versus open surgery for rectal cancer (COLOR II): short term outcomes of randomized, phase 3 trial. Lancet Oncol. 2013;1493:210–8.
8. Keane CR, O'Grady G, Bissett IP, Hayes JL, Hulme-Moir M, Eglinton TW, et al. Functional outcome of laparoscopic-assisted resection versus open resection of rectal cancer: a secondary analysis of the Australasian laparoscopic cancer of the rectum trial. Dis Colon Rectum. 2022;65(7):e698–706.
9. Montori A, de Anna L, Masoni L. Integrated anastomosis using the Knight and Griffen technique. G Chir. 1990;11(3):101–2.
10. Rogers P, Garoufalia Z, Emile SH, Ray-Offor E, Strassmann V, Wexner SD. Optimizing the safety of laparoscopic anterior resection: our approach. Color Dis. 2023;25:2269–70. https://doi.org/10.1111/codi.16747.
11. Salerno G, Sinnatamby C, Branagan G, Daniels IR, Heald RJ, Moran BJ. Defining the rectum: surgically, radiologically, and anatomically. Color Dis. 2006;8(Suppl 3):5–9.
12. Horvat N, Carlos Tavares Rocha C, Clemente Oliveira B, Petkovska I, Gollub MJ. MRI of rectal cancer: tumor staging, imaging techniques, and management. Radiographics. 2019;39(2):367–87.
13. Abramson DJ. The valves of Houston in adults. Am J Surg. 1978;136(3):334–6.
14. Antoniou SA, Huo B, Tzanis AA, Koutsiouroumpa O, Mavridis D, Balla A, Dore S, Kaiser AM, Koraki E, Massey L, Pellino G, Psichogiou M, Sayers AE, Smart NJ, Sylla P, Tschudin-Sutter S, Woodfield JC, Carrano FM, Ortenzi M, Morales-Conde S. EAES, SAGES, and ESCP rapid guideline: bowel preparation for minimally invasive colorectal resection. Surg Endosc. 2023;37(12):9001–12.
15. Rondelli F, Pasculli A, De Rosa M, Avenia S, Bugiantella W. Is routine splenic flexure mobilization always necessary in laparotomic or laparoscopic anterior rectal resection? A systematic review and comprehensive meta-analysis. Updates Surg. 2021;73(5):1643–61.
16. Emile SH, Gilshtein H, Wexner SD. Quadruple assessment of colorectal anastomoses: a technique to reduce the incidence of anastomotic leakage. Color Dis. 2020;22(1):102–3.
17. Martellucci J, Sturiale A, Bergamini C, Boni L, Cianchi F, Coratti A, Valeri A. Role of transanal irrigation in the treatment of anterior resection syndrome. Tech Coloproctol. 2018;22(7):519–27.
18. Battersby NJ, Bouliotis G, Emmertsen KJ, Juul T, Glynne-Jones R, Branagan G, Christensen P, Laurberg S, Moran BJ, UK and Danish LARS Study Groups. Development and external validation of a nomogram and online tool to predict bowel dysfunction following restorative rectal cancer resection: the POLARS score. Gut. 2018;67(4):688–96.

19. Coxon-Meggy AH, Vogel I, White J, Croft J, Corrigan N, Meggy A, et al. Pathway of low anterior resection syndrome relief after surgery (POLARiS) feasibility trial protocol: a multicentre, feasibility cohort study with embedded randomised control trial to compare sacral neuromodulation and transanal irrigation to optimised conservative management in the management of major low anterior resection syndrome following rectal cancer treatment. BMJ Open. 2023;13(1):e064248.

Chapter 6
Laparoscopic Abdominoperineal Resection

Emeka Ray-Offor, Nir Horesh, and Sameh Hany Emile

Introduction

Abdominoperineal resection (APR) was first described in 1908 by Ernest Miles [1]. This procedure involves the removal of the distal colon, rectum, and anal sphincter complex using both anterior abdominal and perineal incisions, resulting in a permanent colostomy. Traditionally, APR was considered the standard treatment of low rectal and anal canal cancers based upon the emphasis on the principle of 5 cm distal clearance of distal spread of the tumor. However, in recent times there has been a decline in the rate of APR for patients diagnosed with distal rectal cancer with the advent of total mesorectal excision (TME), neoadjuvant therapies, and sphincter-saving surgical options. The fundamental concept of TME is based upon the embryology and anatomy of the rectum and the knowledge that rectal cancer is unlikely to spread distally in the muscle tube [2]. APR remains a treatment option in the

---

E. Ray-Offor (✉)
College of Health Sciences, University of Port Harcourt, Choba, Rivers State, Nigeria

Colorectal/Minimal Access Surgery Unit, Department of Surgery University of Port Harcourt Teaching Hospital, Port Harcourt, Rivers State, Nigeria
e-mail: emeka.ray-offor@uniport.edu.ng

N. Horesh
Colorectal Surgery Department, Ellen Leifer Shulman and Steven Shulman Digestive Disease Institute, Cleveland Clinic Florida, Weston, FL, USA

Faculty of Medicine, Tel Aviv University, Tel Aviv, Israel

S. H. Emile
Colorectal Surgery Department, Ellen Leifer Shulman and Steven Shulman Digestive Disease Institute, Cleveland Clinic Florida, Weston, FL, USA

Department of General Surgery, Faculty of Medicine, Mansoura University, Mansoura, Egypt

Schmidt College of Medicine, Florida Atlantic University, Boca Raton, FL, USA

© The Author(s), under exclusive license to Springer Nature Switzerland AG 2024
E. Ray-Offor, R. J. Rosenthal (eds.), *Colorectal & Hernia Laparoscopic Surgery*, https://doi.org/10.1007/978-3-031-63490-1_6

surgeon's toolbox with modifications of the extent of resection designed to yield a cylindrical specimen with an improved circumferential resection margin [3, 4].

Since the introduction of laparoscopic colorectal surgery in 1991, minimally invasive techniques have also been applied to APR [5]. It is noteworthy that several comparative studies between open, laparoscopic, and robotic proctectomy on the pathological outcomes of proctectomy showed similar outcomes [6–9]. However, reduced length of hospital stays and wound infection rates were in favor of minimally invasive surgery. The perineal extraction of specimens which is made possible during APR obviates the need for large abdominal incisions, resulting in significantly reduced post-operative pain. APR is a radical surgery that is likely to be associated with significant comorbidity and potential mortality, hence, calls for appropriate patient selection and adequate surgical expertise.

Relevant Anatomy

The rectum is the most distal part of the large intestine measuring about 12 centimeters in length. This terminal segment of the bowel along with the anal canal has unique features as described in Chap. 5. To guide surgical management, rectal cancers are traditionally categorized based on distance from the anal verge into the upper, mid, and low rectal. Low rectal cancers, located <6 cm from the anal verge, are usually indicated for APR. It is noteworthy that the external anal sphincter has a variable length and angulation at the puborectalis hence height above the anal verge is variable. Hence it is more apt to use the distance of the tumor from the external anal sphincter to render the decision on APR. In patients with rectal tumors and incontinence for APR to improve quality of life, the decision for the surgery needs to be made after clinical and DRE evaluation of the sphincters.

The pelvic diaphragm (levator ani) consists of the puborectalis muscle which blends with the top of the external sphincter forming the anorectal ring, palpable posteriorly on digital rectal examination. In addition, muscle fibers posterior to the puborectalis sweep backward onto the pelvic surface of iliococcygeus and are inserted onto the front of the coccyx and the anococcygeal raphe, to form the pubococcygeus muscle (Fig. 6.1). The other component muscle of the pelvic diaphragm is the coccygeus muscle.

In the standard APR, the resected specimen is coned down by resection of the levator ani muscles closer to the rectum— the 'waist' effect. This has a potential risk of circumferential involvement of tumour cells. The modifications of the extra levator and beyond-levator APR techniques emphasize the relationship between the tumor and the circumferential margin. A cylindrical specimen is achieved by a broader resection of the levator muscle for an R0 resection. An extension of the perineal resection margin to incorporate most of the ischiorectal fossa is done in the beyond-levator APR technique.

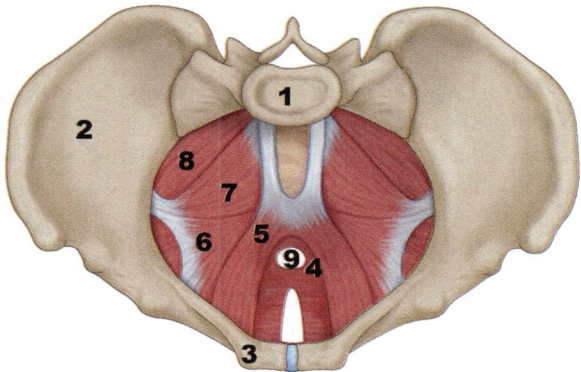

Fig. 6.1 Superior view of pelvic floor: (1) Sacrum; (2) Iliac bone; (3) Pubic bone; (4) Puborectalis; (5) Pubococcygeus; (6) Iliococcygeus; (7) Ischiococcygeus; (8) Piriformis; (9) Anorectal hiatus (Adapted from pelvic floor www.shutterstock.com)

Indications

Malignant

APR is indicated in ultra-low rectal tumors within 5 cm of the anal verge when it is not possible to achieve a negative distal margin (5 cm proximally and 2 cm distally), involvement of the external sphincter or invasion of the levator ani complex. In addition, the procedure should be considered in patients with significant incontinence who would benefit from a permanent colostomy [10]. This radical surgery aims to remove the tumor, associated lymphoid tissue, and involved structures from within the deep pelvis. A critical balance in decision-making is required in choosing between APR and sphincter-saving surgery for low rectal cancers. Sphincter-saving surgery would preserve bowel continuity but at the expense of poor functional outcome and low anterior resection syndrome (LARS) whereas APR would avoid this adverse outcome yet with increased risk of local recurrence, perineal hernia, pelvic collection, and loss of normal bowel continuity.

Patients with anal cancers with failure of preoperative CRT or who experience recurrence after CRT are also offered APR.

Benign

Specific inflammatory bowel disease patients are candidates for APR. These include Crohn's proctitis with anal disease and ulcerative colitis patients who are not candidates for ileal pouch-anal anastomoses (IPAA) [11]. Other benign indications are fecal incontinence not amenable to sphincter-sparing surgery and extensive Fournier's gangrene [12].

Contraindications

Patients who are unfit for general anesthesia are not offered a major resection surgery like APR. Relative contraindications include those at high risk of poor postoperative outcomes such as poorly controlled diabetes, morbid obesity, frailty, and immunosuppression.

Preoperative Preparation

Relevant clinical evaluation of a patient is required based on the patient's age and overall medical condition. These include routine laboratory investigations consisting of a full blood count, chemistry, grouping, and cross-matching. Cardiopulmonary risk is assessed by ECG and chest radiography. All patients undergo preoperative stoma site marking and education. This service is offered by the surgeon or preferably a stoma therapist. The future colostomy site should be marked to avoid possible bony prominence, scars, natural skin folds, and conversion midline incision. Usually, patients receive a mechanical bowel preparation in addition to oral antibiotics comprising oral neomycin or erythromycin and metronidazole to reduce postoperative surgical site infection. Parenteral antibiotic prophylaxis comprising a first-generation cephalosporin with metronidazole is administered within 30 minutes of incision. Compression devices are applied to the calves for deep vein thrombosis prophylaxis and the full ERAS protocol is instituted [13]. A theatre consult invitation can be extended to the Urology and Reconstructive surgery team for specialist service as anticipated for surgery.

The OR equipment for advanced laparoscopic surgery which comprises monitor screens, gas insufflator, camera scope (10 mm, 30-degree angled scope), laparoscopic instruments, endoscopic linear stapler, and advanced sealing devices (Harmonic, LigaSure) are prechecked.

Anesthesia

General anesthesia with endotracheal intubation is required.

Positioning

The patient is carefully positioned in modified lithotomy in a hydraulic stirrup with less hip flexion to allow uninhibited dissection along the left colic gutter. Great care is taken to carefully pad and protect all areas of potential pressure injury and the patient is secured onto the table with a strap across the chest.

Technique

The anus, perineum, and vagina are prepped and draped in the usual sterile manner. Cystoscopy with placement of bilateral ureteric catheters is performed by the urologist.

A digital rectal examination is done to reconfirm the site of the lesion relative to the anal verge and sphincter complex. A mushroom-tipped catheter is placed in the rectum through which approximately 1 L of normal saline is irrigated until the effluent is clear. Betadine solution is then introduced into the catheter which has its end connected to a plastic urine bag. The catheter is then removed after drainage of the introduced fluid.

A sequential one or two-team approach is herein described. An infraumbilical vertical incision is made and carefully extended into the peritoneum to introduce a 10-mm Hasson cannula. Carbon dioxide pneumoperitoneum of 12–15 mmHg is achieved after which a 30-degree telescope is carefully introduced. Four or five trocars may be used: a 10-mm umbilical trocar for a 30-degree laparoscope, 10-mm and 5-mm trocars in the right lower quadrant and upper quadrants for most of the dissection respectively, and at least one additional left lower quadrant 5-mm port for the assistant to provide retraction. A diagnostic laparoscopy is then performed after trocar placement to assess for metastatic disease. The liver surface is inspected, and intraoperative ultrasound may be used, if available. The small bowel, peritoneal surfaces, and periaortic nodes are inspected in addition to an assessment of the resectability of the pelvic mass. If adjudged unresectable due to locally advanced disease or widespread metastases, the patient may be better served by palliative diversion alone.

With a combination of right side down and head down, dissection is started laterally at the junction between the descending and sigmoid colons and mobilizing medially and cephalad in the plane anterior to Gerota fascia and retroperitoneum as described in LAR (Chap. 5) the entire left colon is carefully mobilized using 10-mm diameter Babcock grasping forceps, 5-mm diameter Harmonic scalpel. The left and right ureters should be identified throughout the dissection to avoid injury. The inferior mesenteric artery is then located between the aorta and the left colic artery and is carefully divided following an incision into the mesentery distal to the outline of the vasculature with an advanced bipolar sealing device e.g., 10 mm LigaSure Atlas. Similarly, the inferior mesenteric vein is located at the left lateral border of the duodenum at the inferior margin of the pancreas above the level of the left colic vein and is similarly divided. The mesentery is divided to the level of the middle colic vessels; in addition, the mesentery is divided from the level of ligation of the artery to the level of the sigmoid-descending junction. The sigmoid-descending junction is then carefully transected with a single 60-mm endoscopic linear cutting stapler firing using a purple cartridge.

The dissection is then continued down to the pelvis along the areolar layer between the fascia propria of the rectum and the presacral fascia from the level of the sacral promontory. Care must be taken at this point to identify and preserve the hypogastric nerves. The posterior dissection is continued down to the level of the levator muscles. The lateral ligaments should be divided as close as possible to the specimen without compromising the radial margins to avoid injury to the nervi erigentes. With the division of the lateral stalks bilaterally, attention is then shifted anteriorly. With downward traction on the rectum and upward traction with a retractor on the vagina or prostate, the rectovaginal septum is dissected in women, or the layer posterior to Denonvilliers' fascia in men down to the pelvic floor anteriorly. When the pelvic floor is reached circumferentially around the rectum, the abdominal portion of the dissection is completed.

From the perineum, the anus is again prepped, then effaced with a Lone Star retractor. The anus is sutured shut with 2 concentric #0 silk purse string suture (Fig. 6.2). An elliptical incision is created and is extended from the midpoint of the perineal body in males, or the posterior vaginal introitus in females back to a point midway between the coccyx and the anus. Wider margins on the perianal skin are taken for lower lesions (Fig. 6.3).

Using electrocautery, dissection is started posteriorly and is advanced laterally and then anteriorly. Great care is taken not to injure the vagina. However, an anteriorly based tumor in women may necessitate an excision of a cuff of the posterior vaginal wall. For an extra levator APR, a wide circumferential incision of the levator muscle is done (Fig. 6.4). The resection specimen is extracted through the perineum. Afterward, copious irrigation is done, and meticulous hemostasis is assured. The perineal wound is closed in layers. When sufficient levator muscle remains, the

Fig. 6.2 Effaced purse-string sutured anal canal

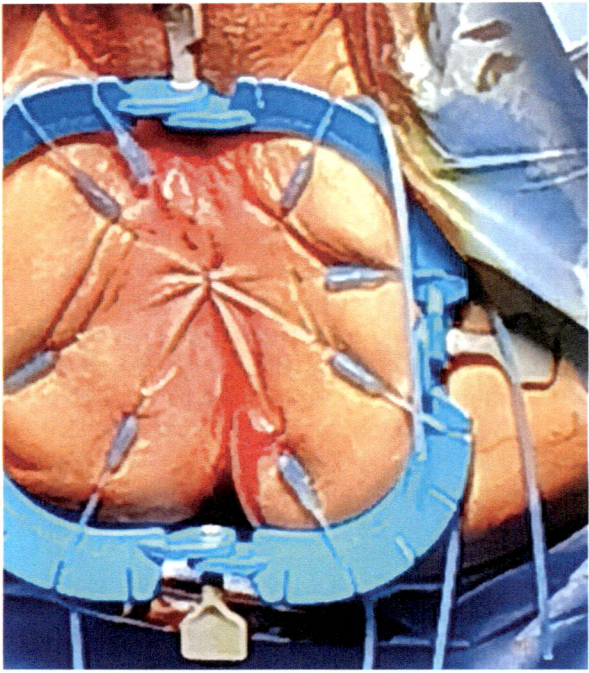

Fig. 6.3 Elliptical perianal incision

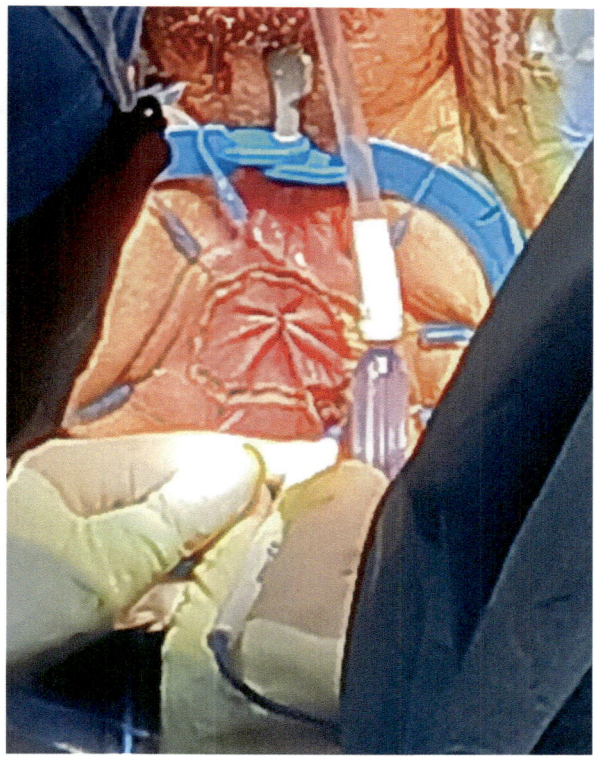

Fig. 6.4 Securing hemostasis in perineal defect following abdominoperineal excision

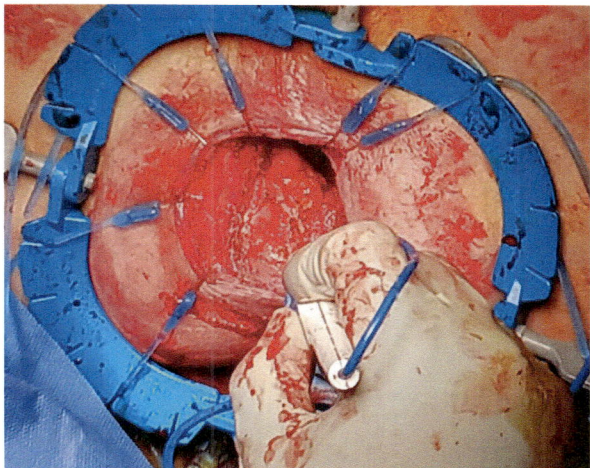

pelvic floor is reapproximated with multiple absorbable sutures. A closed drain is inserted below the reapproximated levator muscles, exiting laterally in the perineum. The skin is reapproximated using interrupted permanent monofilament suture in a

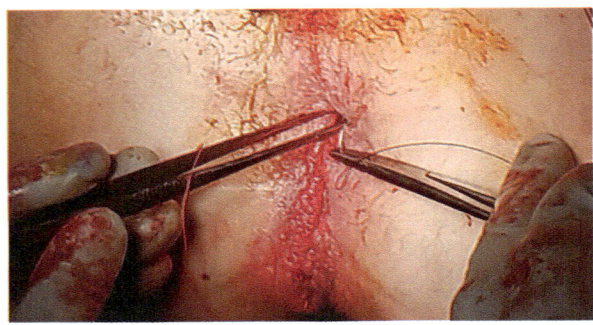

Fig. 6.5 Skin closure of perineal wound

vertical mattress fashion (Fig. 6.5). With insufficient levator muscle, repair of the perineal defect by the reconstructive surgery team with a planned vertical rectus abdominus myocutaneous flap closure is warranted. Simple suture approximation of the subcutaneous fat in the ischiorectal space in the midline may be done using interrupted absorbable sutures, however, there is an increased risk for perineal herniation. The use of biological/dual mesh or omentoplasty for perineal wound closure after APR is reported with no clear consensus on the "best" option, and tailoring to the individual remains a critical factor [14].

The abdomen is insufflated and after further irrigation and verification of meticulous hemostasis, a 19 mm Blake drain is placed through a stab wound in the right lower quadrant, left to rest in the presacral space, and sutured to skin with 2-0 Prolene. The previously identified left-sided colostomy site is re-identified and a 2-cm disk of skin is excised. A 10 mm port is placed through the colostomy site and the descending colon is gently grasped. The anaesthesiologist administers 3.5 mL of indocyanine green and a 10 mL flush to establish excellent perfusion at the intended area for the colostomy. The underlying fat and anterior rectus sheath is incised in the cephalad to caudad direction. The rectus fibers are spread along their axis and the posterior sheath and peritoneum are incised in a cephalad to caudad direction. The colon is delivered through the stoma site so that 5 cm rests above the skin in a tension-free manner. After further irrigation and assurance of hemostasis, the abdomen is desufflated and port sites are closed. Dry dressings are applied to the abdominal port and perineal surgical sites. The stoma is then primarily matured as described in Chap. 2. An appliance is placed over the healthy pink, well-vented stoma, and the patient is transferred to the recovery room in a stable condition.

Post-operative Care

The resected specimen is sent to the Pathology laboratory. Early ambulation is advised with patients encouraged out of bed on # 1 postoperative day on adequate analgesia. Oral intake is resumed #1 postoperative day. Broad-spectrum antibiotics are administered for 5–7 days. With the commencement of stoma function the drain is removed, and the patient is discharged home. The perineal sutures are kept in place following extra levator APR for at least 2 weeks to allow ample time for healing, especially if the patient received neoadjuvant radiation therapy. Postoperative cancer surveillance is conducted according to the NCCN guidelines [15]. Procedure-specific complications of APR are categorized into nerve injury, urologic injury, perineal wound, and ostomy-related complications [16].

Peroneal nerve injury may result from incorrect stirrup use; hence careful attention should be paid to patient positioning. Shoulder padding helps prevent brachial plexus injury in a steep Trendelenburg position. In addition, sexual and urinary function may be compromised during pelvic dissection after injury of the autonomic nerves. In men, sexual dysfunction is recognizable as the inability to achieve erection, partial erection, or retrograde ejaculation [17].

Iatrogenic or direct tumor invasion-related urologic injuries may result. Sound surgical technique involves clear identification of the ureters and their exclusion from the dissection field. When an injury is identified during surgery, a primary repair over a stent is indicated. Bladder injuries require a double row of interrupted suture repair with polyglactin suture. The urethral catheter should ideally be retained for 10–14 days after urologic injuries.

The need for a permanent colostomy invites a peculiar set of complications that may occur in the immediate setting or the long term. The management of some of these complications has been addressed in Chap. 2 of this book.

Multiple perineal wound complications may occur after APR, including infection, breakdown, sinus, and delayed healing. The incidence of perineal wound complications after APR can range from 26 to 41% [18]. A report suggests that the perineal wound complication rate is about twice as high in patients treated with cylindrical APR than in those treated with conventional APR. [19] Perineal hernias can occur in up to 13% of cases of intersphincteric APR but rise to 25% of cases in extended resections including the sphincters [19].

References

1. Miles WE. A method of performing abdominoperineal excision for carcinoma of the rectum and of the terminal portion of the pelvic colon (1908). CA Cancer J Clin. 1971;21:361–4.
2. MacFarlane JK, Ryall RD, Heald RJ. Mesorectal excision for rectal cancer. Lancet. 1993;341(8843):457–60.
3. Bianco F, Romano G, Tsarkov P, Stanojevic G, Shroyer K, Giuratrabocchetta S, Bergamaschi R, International Rectal Cancer Study Group. Extralevator with vs nonextralevator abdominoperineal excision for rectal cancer: the RELAPe randomized controlled trial. Color Dis. 2017;19:148–57.
4. Seshadri RA, West NP, Sundersingh S. A pilot randomized study comparing extralevator with conventional abdominoperineal excision for low rectal cancer after neoadjuvant chemoradiation. Color Dis. 2017;19:O253–62.
5. Jacobs M, Verdeja JC, Goldstein HS. Minimally invasive colon resection (laparoscopic colectomy). Surg Laparosc Endosc. 1991;1:144–50.
6. Kitaguchi D, Tsukada Y, Ito M, Horasawa S, Bando H, Yoshino T, Yamada K, Ajioka Y, Sugihara K. Survival outcomes following salvage abdominoperineal resection for recurrent and persistent anal squamous cell carcinoma. Eur J Surg Oncol. 2023;49:106929. S0748-7983(23)00488-2.

7. Garfinkle R, Abou-Khalil M, Bhatnagar S, Wong-Chong N, Azoulay L, Morin N, et al. A comparison of pathological outcomes of open, laparoscopic and robotic resections for rectal cancer using ACS-NSQIP proctectomy-targeted database: a propensity score analysis. J Gastrointest Surg. 2019;23(2):348–56.
8. Bedrikovetsi S, Dudi-Venkata NN, Kroon HM, Moore JW, Hunter RA, Sammour T. Outcomes of minimally invasive versus open proctectomy for rectal cancer: a propensity-matched analysis of bi-national colorectal cancer audit data. Dis Colon Rectum. 2020;63(6):778–87.
9. Zhang GQ, Sahyoun R, Stem M, Lo BD, Rajput A, Efron JE, et al. Operative approach does not impact radial margin positivity in distal rectal cancer. World J Surg. 2021;45(12):3686–94.
10. Garcia-Henriquez N, Galante DJ, Monson JRT. Selection and outcomes in abdominoperineal resection. Front Oncol. 2020;10:1339.
11. Meima-van Praag EM, Buskens CJ, Hompes R, Bemelman WA. Surgical management of Crohn's disease: a state-of-the-art review. Int J Color Dis. 2021;36(6):1133–45.
12. Holden J, Nayak JG, Botkin C, Helewa RM. Abdominoperineal resection with absorbable mesh repair of perineal defect for Fournier's gangrene: a case report. Int Med Case Rep J. 2021;14:133–8.
13. Gustafsson UO, Scott MJ, Schwenk W, Demartines N, Roulin D, Francis N, et al.; Enhanced Recovery After Surgery Society. Guidelines for perioperative care in elective colonic surgery: enhanced recovery after surgery (ERAS®) society recommendations. Clin Nutr. 2012;31(6):783–800.
14. Riva CG, Kelly ME, Vitellaro M, Rottoli M, Aiolfi A, Ferrari D, et al. A comparison of surgical techniques for perineal wound closure following perineal excision: a systematic review and network meta-analysis. Tech Coloproctol. 2023;27(12):1351–66.
15. Benson AB, Venook AP, Al-Hawary MM, Azad N, Chen YJ, Ciombor KK, et al. Rectal cancer, version 2.2022, NCCN clinical practice guidelines in oncology. J Natl Compr Cancer Netw. 2022;20(10):1139–67.
16. Perry WB, Connaughton JC. Abdominoperineal resection: how is it done and what are the results? Clin Colon Rectal Surg. 2007;20(3):213–20.
17. Artioukh DY, Smith RA, Gokul K. Risk factors for impaired healing of the perineal wound after abdominoperineal resection of rectum for carcinoma. Color Dis. 2007;9:362–7.
18. Bullard KM, Trudel JL, Baxter NN, et al. Primary perineal wound closure after preoperative radiotherapy and abdominoperineal resection has a high incidence of wound failure. Dis Colon Rectum. 2005;48:438–43.
19. Christian CK, Kwaan MR, Betensky RA, et al. Risk factors for perineal wound complications following abdominoperineal resection. Dis Colon Rectum. 2005;48:43–8.

Chapter 7
Laparoscopic Restorative Proctectomy with Ileal Pouch-Anal Anastomosis

Olusegun Komolafe

Introduction

Restorative proctectomy (RP) was described in 1978 by Alan Parks and John Nicholls [1]. This surgical procedure involves the creation of a pelvic ileal reservoir in continuity with the anal canal following the surgical removal of the colon and rectum. A permanent stoma is avoided which improves the patient's quality of life. RP has evolved from the original description which involved mucosectomy and hand-sewn anastomosis, to a straightforward double-stapled anastomosis with a better functional outcome [2, 3]. A J-shaped pouch configuration is frequently performed compared to earlier reports of S-shaped and W-shaped configurations [4].

Controversies in ileal pouch surgery include the choice of diversion or not, the timing of biologic therapy, and the outcome of surgery in obesity, and the elderly [4]. Minimally invasive surgery, employing either laparoscopic, robotic, or transanal laparoscopic approaches, is currently the preferred approach in the elective setting. A reduction in length of hospital stay, blood transfusion, post-operative gastrointestinal disorders, and septicemia is reported when compared to the open approach, though the laparoscopic approach can take a longer time to perform.

A good knowledge of potential pitfalls in the early peri-operative period, and long-term challenges following RP is required of surgeons performing this surgery as these have immense implications on patients. There is a need for careful patient selection.

O. Komolafe (✉)
University Hospital Wishaw, Wishaw, Scotland

University of Glasgow, Glasgow, Scotland
e-mail: segun.komolafe@lanarkshire.scot.nhs.uk

Relevant Anatomy

Anatomical considerations for proctectomy in "benign" disease are similar to those for oncological resection. Whilst theoretically feasible to perform an "intra-mesorectal" dissection, hemostasis is difficult in this plane with the potential for more complications. Balanced against this would be a lesser chance of hypogastric nerve injury. Most rectal surgeons are familiar with the TME plane, so it is logical to use this in this scenario.

The other major anatomical consideration is small bowel mobility: the distal ileum needs to reach the pelvic floor, to allow the formation of a J-pouch. This should be assessed early during the procedure, as occasionally, it may be physically impossible to form a tension-free ileal pouch-anal anastomosis, such as in a patient with short, fatty mesentery, or if there have been intra-abdominal adhesions.

Indications and Contraindications

In simplest terms, any patient without a rectum and colon can be considered for an IPAA. This tends to be patients in two broad categories: those undergoing procto-colectomy for inflammatory bowel disease (IBD), or for colonic polyposis. Surgery for UC is indicated in medically refractory patients, failure to tolerate medical treatment or its adverse effects, and in the presence of coexisting neoplastic or dysplastic transformation of the intestinal mucosa [5–7].

Generally, patients with Crohn's disease should not be offered IPAA, for the obvious reason that both the terminal ileum and anal canal are affected by Crohn's. However, some surgeons do offer IPAA to a select population of CD patients with no history of peri-anal or small bowel disease after proper pre-operative counseling. CD has a five-fold higher risk of failure, and a two-fold risk of strictures after IPAA compared with UC. The function in those who retain the pouch is reported to be similar to that of patients with UC [8–10]. Indeterminate colitis and primary sclerosing cholangitis are other relative contraindications to IPAA as patients with these conditions are associated with high post-operative morbidity. When there is a cancerous lesion in the distal rectum, requiring an abdominoperineal resection, or there is an incompetent anal sphincter mechanism, or in emergency presentation with accompanying use of high-dose steroid, IPAA should not be considered.

Pre-operative Preparation

A review of all colonic biopsies, and previous colectomy specimens where there is one, as well as confirmation, with the attending Pathologist in the IBD MDT that there is no misdiagnosis of Crohn's Colitis is made. This is particularly pertinent when a patient has "Indeterminate" colitis, as a proportion of these patients have unproven Crohn's colitis and are likely to have a poor outcome from IPAA.

If it is anticipated that the patient will have good pelvic floor/sphincter function, and there are no oncological concerns, the main decision-making hinges on the patient's quality of life (QoL) expectations and preferences. To help patients with this, anticipated outcomes, including complications, and short-, medium- and long-term issues should be walked through with the patient, and this may require more than one consultation. Patients can also be directed to accurate online platforms, to discuss with other patients. It is the author's practice to point the prospective patient to other patients with IPAA, who have agreed to act as patient counselors, for a local, age-relevant context.

Patients with any Mendelian disorder (Familial Adenomatous Polyposis, Lynch Syndrome, etc.), undergoing risk reduction surgery, need specific counseling as they are going from a "normal" situation to a significant change in bowel function with a pouch. This is distinctive from UC patients who have had pain, diarrhea, and haematochezia, with a failure of medical therapies, and therefore have different QoL expectations. Some patients with genetic abnormalities may only be identified as such, during diagnosis of colonic or rectal cancer, so are undergoing both an oncological, and prophylactic, procedure. Patients undergoing proctectomy do not need any bowel preparation.

Pouches and Pregnancy

Several challenges are associated with pouches and pregnancy, and patients must be managed in a multi-disciplinary manner involving Obstetrics, Gastroenterology, and Surgery, particularly as there is a paucity of robust scientific data [11, 12]. Females of childbearing age need prior counseling on reduced fertility following surgery involving the pelvis, especially if they run into any complications. There is some evidence that reduced fertility may also correlate with pre-operative disease severity [13]. They will also need counseling about pregnancy, and the effects of mode of delivery on their (future) pouch function. Some patients who have had emergent total colectomy will opt to defer completion of proctectomy and IPAA until after their family is complete.

Pouch continence may be compromised by vaginal delivery, especially a prolonged second stage of labor; and also, by perineal injuries or episiotomies. However, some pouch patients can have a vaginal delivery with reasonable pouch function, even after instrumental vaginal delivery [14]. The appropriate delivery route should be decided on a case-by-case basis within MDT to ensure safe delivery for mother and child without compromising pouch function. It is reasonable to ensure experienced Obstetricians, and Colorectal Surgeons, are readily available for elective, and emergent deliveries for pouch patients.

Anesthesia

Enhanced Recovery After Surgery principles are well-established for patients undergoing major colorectal procedures.

Positioning, Access, Trocar Placement

The patient is positioned in the low Lloyd-Davis position, for an anterior resection, as previously discussed (Chap. 5), however after positioning, the two proctectomy procedures require a slightly different set-up.

Completion Proctectomy + IPAA: The patient will have scars from a previous colectomy, as well as an ileostomy. Scars from incisions and ports should be avoided for safe access. Access will be sequential as adhesions within the peritoneum may have to be taken down to allow safe port placement. The first port for a camera can be a 5 mm or 12 mm port according to the available camera size. The next port will be a working port for an energy device to take down adhesions, with further ports as then safely possible.

One option is to take down the ileostomy, and then use the Alexis retractor with a trocar inserted through the lid to establish and maintain the pneumo-peritoneum. Further ports can be inserted so that there can be triangulation on the pelvis—similar to the standard setup for an anterior resection (Fig. 7.1). A subtle but important issue is to ensure that the working ports are medial enough to reach the pelvic floor, especially in the narrow male pelvis.

A second option is to leave the stoma intact and gain access through an optical port in the left upper quadrant. A further port is inserted in the left iliac fossa, then a midline umbilical port, with a final port in the right iliac fossa. This is similar to port placements for a right hemicolectomy (Fig. 7.2).

Pan-Proctocolectomy + IPAA: Port placements will be for a total colectomy (TC), ensuring that the working ports are slightly medial to reach the pelvic floor, essentially ports in all four quadrants, with the LUQ and RIF working ports being 12 mm ports so that the preferred energy device, a LigaSure Atlas® can be used for dissection (Fig. 7.3).

Total Colectomy: Steps are as described elsewhere for segmental colectomy (Chap. 3). The sequence can vary according to surgical preference. The author's preference is to start the dissection at the left pelvic brim with the sigmoid colon, then progress proximally to terminal ileum TI which must be mobilized completely off the pelvic brim. The author also preferentially uses a 10 mm laparoscopic energy device (LigaSure Atlas®) which allows quicker division of the mesocolon, and better haemostasis around the flexures and gastro-colic omentum.

Proctectomy: For patients undergoing pan-proctocolectomy, dissection is a distal extension of the prior sigmoid mobilization, entering the TME plane behind the inferior mesenteric artery (IMA)/superior haemorrhoidal artery (SHA). For patients

7 Laparoscopic Restorative Proctectomy with Ileal Pouch-Anal Anastomosis

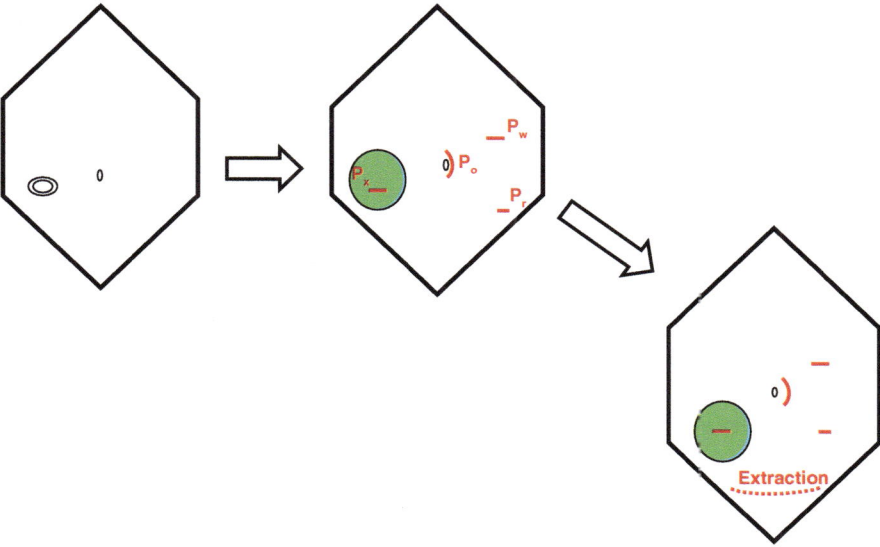

Fig. 7.1 Port placement for Laparoscopic Completion Proctectomy with Ileostomy site for first access: P_o—12 mm Optical Port, P_w—12 mm Working instrument port, P_x—12 mm Working instrument port in Alexis® retractor, P_r—5 mm Retracting instrument port

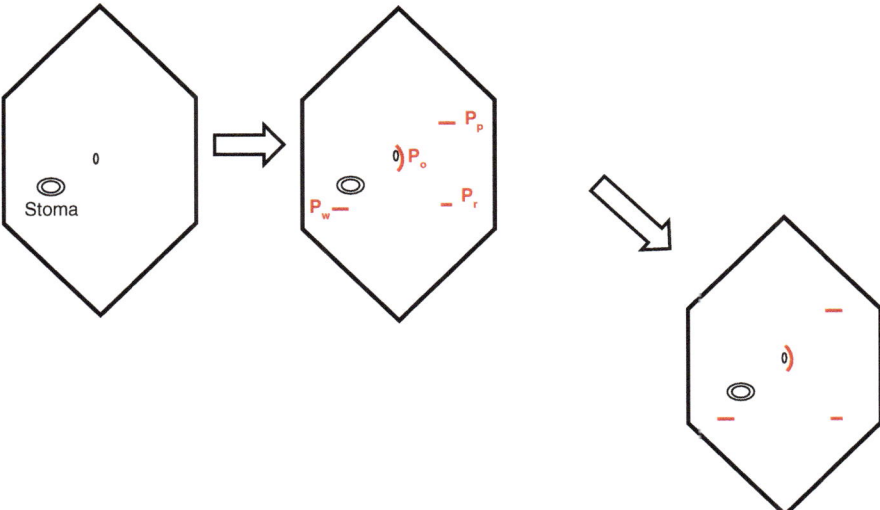

Fig. 7.2 Port placement for Lap Completion Proctectomy with Palmer's point/Left upper quadrant for first access: P_o—12 mm Optical Port, P_w—12 mm Working instrument port, P_x—12 mm Working instrument port in Alexis® retractor, P_r—5 mm Retracting instrument port. Stoma taken down after division of recto-anal junction, then J-pouch fashioned through extraction wound

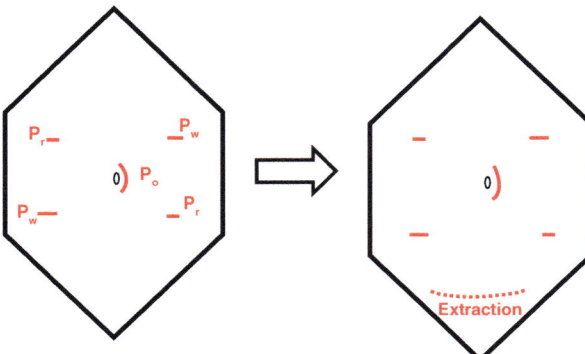

Fig. 7.3 Port placement for Laparoscopic Pan-proctocolectomy: P_o—12 mm Optical Port, P_w—12 mm Working instrument port, P_r—5 mm Retracting instrument port

undergoing CP, dissection begins by identification of the rectal stump, and then attempting to dissect posterior to the stump to enter the TME plane. If the SHA has been spared at the prior TC, ligating the vessel and dissecting the posterior will lead to the correct plane with the mesorectal fascia intact. The pelvic dissection in IBD can be made difficult as the rectum is inflamed, so there can be prominent mesorectal nodes, increased vascularity, and "sticky" planes with the embryological planes of cleavage not always clearly defined.

TME proctectomy is described elsewhere, and the steps are standard, mobilizing the rectum down to the pelvic floor circumferentially. The author's practice is to perform EUA before proctectomy and inject 1–2 mL of methylene blue into the anal wall just above the dentate line, in the anterior and posterior midline. This brings certainty that the laparoscopic dissection has reached the anal canal, when the methylene blue blush is identified in the anterior and posterior bowel, marking the distal limit of dissection, and anorectal vascularity is confirmed at this point with ICG. A Pfannenstiel incision is made, and the anorectal junction is divided with a single firing of the Contour® stapler, after again confirming the limit of dissection with the digit.

Ileal Pouch Formation and Pouch-Anal Anastomosis: The Pfannenstiel incision allows delivery of the colon and rectum, and division of TI, usually with another firing of the Contour stapler. TI is doubled back on itself to form a J-shaped loop of bowel, with the apex of the J reaching the pubic tubercle comfortably. Surgical lore is that a loop of bowel that reaches the symphysis pubis comfortably will similarly reach the pelvic floor for anastomosis. The length of the J-pouch can be between 15 and 20 cm. ICG is used to check there are no issues with ileal vascularity, then an enterotomy is made in the apex, and the pouch is fashioned with two firings of a 100 mm linear stapler.

The apical enterotomy is closed over the anvil of a circular stapler, with a purse string—the author's practice is a "double" purse string to ensure the proximal bowel is securely tied around the anvil. The pouch apex is returned to the abdomen, and the pneumo-peritoneum is re-established, for intra-corporeal anastomosis, as it can be difficult to see the upper anal canal staple line properly at open surgery. The circular stapler is brought through the anus very carefully, and the spike passed through the staple line, to dock with the pouch anvil. Both sides of the joint are brought together, with a third and final infusion of ICG to check vascularity on both sides. The stapler can then be fired, and anastomosis assessed with the digit. A flexible sigmoidoscope is inserted to check for any staple line air leaks laparoscopically, with the pouch fully submerged under water within the pelvis, and TI proximal to the pouch occluded to prevent proximal gas escape.

Ileostomy: If there are no significant intra-operative concerns, there is no definitive reason for de-functioning ileostomy, as a routine. The author's practice is not to de-function young, patients who have had an unremarkable procedure, with no concerns during or after anastomosis—no staple line leaks, thick circular stapler donuts, good blood supply seen with ICG, no significant blood loss, no co-morbidities, no recent immuno-modulatory drugs. Patients with any of these issues can have a de-functioning loop ileostomy.

It must always be borne in mind that loop ileostomy itself is not without complications [15]. Anecdotally, within the author's cohort of patients, de-functioning loop ileostomies have caused more complications than the pouch-anal anastomoses they were created to protect! If a patient is de-functioned, the ileostomy should be closed as early as possible, typically in 8–12 weeks, so that the de-functioned pouch does not atrophy which reduces its reservoir capacity and can compromise pouch function due to bacterial overgrowth, etc.

Complications

A detailed discussion of pouch complications and management is outside the scope of this chapter; however, it is important to be aware of these [16, 17]. One of the main, and defining, advantages of high-volume units is there should be established pathways and processes, to quickly identify, and rescue, the failing patient. It can be helpful to classify pouch-associated complications, into immediate/short-term, medium-term, and long-term. This certainly helps frame the discussion with patients during pre-operative counseling and consenting.

Immediate: These are peri-operative complications related directly to the procedure, the most significant being stapled line leaks, anastomotic leaks, and pelvic sepsis. These need to be anticipated by rigorous post-op care, and early detection of any deviation from normal physiology. Pouches can be salvaged by early endoscopic (Fig. 7.4), radiological, or surgical interventions for any leaks or sepsis. De-functioned pouches can be easier to manage, due to the absence of the fecal stream. A patient who does not have one may need to be de-functioned, to facilitate management of any pouch complications.

Medium-term:

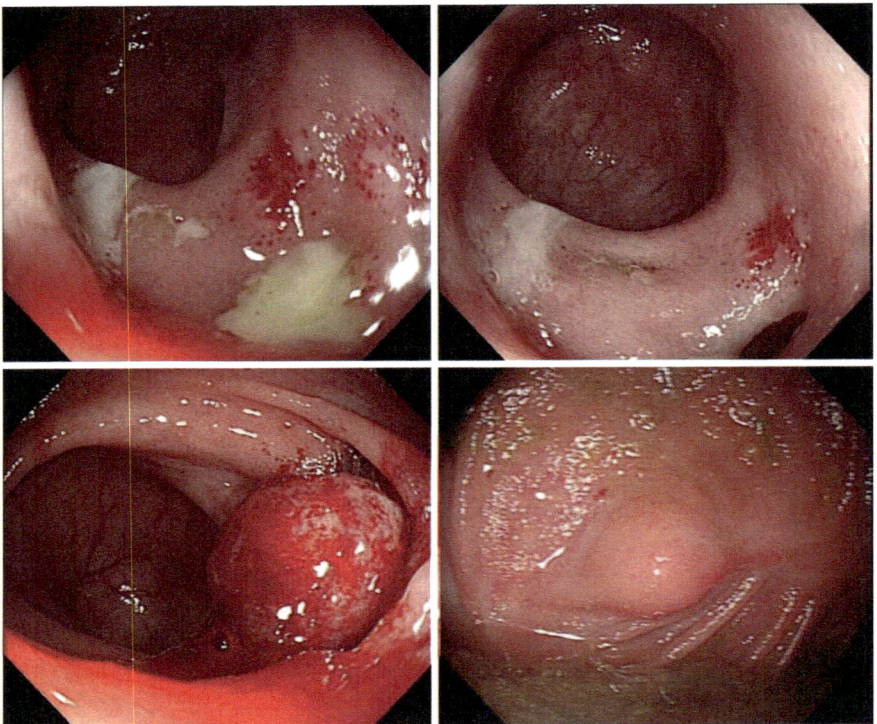

Fig. 7.4 Defect in the pouch staple line closed with Over the scope (OTS) Clip, anti-clockwise from top right: defect identified, purulent discharge from defect, defect closed with OTC clip, defect healed

- Pouchitis is inflammation of the pouch, typically causing over-activity of the pouch, with urgency and diarrhea, occurring in up to 50% of patients at some point [16]. The etiology is not completely understood; however, treatment is with antibiotics suggesting an interplay with the bacterial flora within the pouch. Supporting this is the finding that patients taking live bacteria preparations can have an improvement in their pouch function (Fig. 7.5).
- Some pouch patients have undiagnosed Crohn's disease. These patients then present with peri-anal features of CD—fistulae, abscess, stenosis, and abscesses. They can also develop recalcitrant pouchitis. Such patients will need input from Gastroenterology, and re-commencement of immune-modulatory drugs, with some eventually needed in their pouch explanted.
- UC patients who have not had their bowel divided at the anorectal junction are left with a cuff of the rectum, which can then become inflamed, "cuffitis". This can be managed with topical treatment for UC with suppositories or enemas. Some thought may have to be given to revisional surgery if this is unsuccessful, though this needs to be in expert hands.

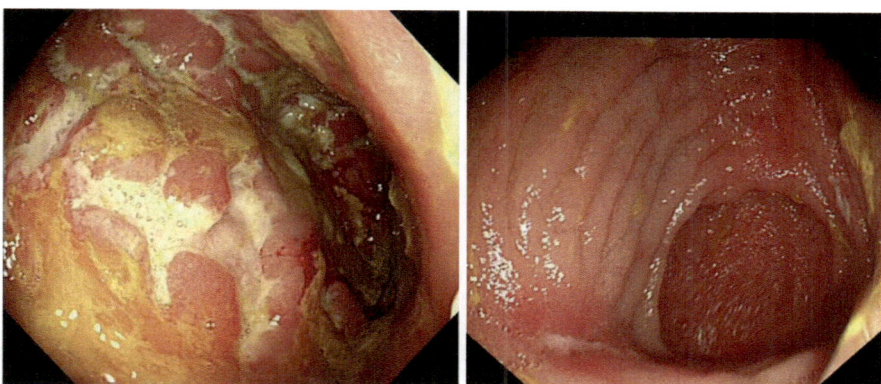

Fig. 7.5 Chronic pouchitis with deep ulcers much improved after alternating anti-biotic courses, with a resolution of symptoms

- Patients may develop problems with pouch evacuation. The pouch needs to be assessed endoscopically and radiologically to ensure no physical cause for this such as anastomotic stenosis, or acuity of the pouch—anus angle related to scarring with time, or other scarring within the pouch which can become dumb-bell shaped, with the proximal chamber not emptying. These can be assessed with flexible pouchoscopy or defecating pouchogram. Cross-sectional imaging can also be helpful, but is not always discriminatory, as it is a dynamic, functional problem.

Long-term: Long-term pouch issues can be related to scarring, resulting in staple line stenoses. Some pouches tend to gradually distend with time, with the potential for bacterial overgrowth, evacuatory difficulties, and chronic pouchitis. Some patients develop "Irritable Pouch Syndrome" with a constellation of pouch-related symptoms, which can be difficult to manage, especially if there are psychosocial contributory factors. A proportion of pouches cease to function well, after years or even decades, for poorly understood reasons, needing explanation.

References

1. Parks AG, Nicholls RJ. Proctocolectomy without ileostomy for ulcerative colitis. Br Med J. 1978;2:85–8.
2. Utsunomiya J, Iwama T, Imajo M, Matsuo S, Sawai S, Yaegashi K, et al. Total colectomy, mucosal proctectomy, and ileoanal anastomosis. Dis Colon Rectum. 1980;23:459–66.
3. Ng KS, Gonsalves SJ, Sagar PM. Ileal-anal pouches: a review of its history, indications, and complications. World J Gastroenterol. 2019;25(31):4320–42.
4. Hull TL, Kiran RP, Stocchi L, Zaghiyan K, Read TE, Hyman NH. Controversies in the ileoanal pouch. J Gastrointest Surg. 2022;25:3019–23.
5. Liu S, Eisenstein S. State-of-the-art surgery for ulcerative colitis. Langenbecks Arch Surg. 2021;406(6):1751–61.

6. Chang S, Shen B, Remzi F. When not to pouch: important considerations for patient selection for ileal pouch-anal anastomosis. Gastroenterol Hepatol (N Y). 2017;13:466–75.
7. McLaughlin SD, Clark SK, Tekkis PP, Ciclitira PJ, Nicholls RJ. Review article: restorative proctocolectomy, indications, management of complications and follow-up—a guide for gastroenterologists. Aliment Pharmacol Ther. 2008;27:895–909.
8. Bemelman WA, Warusavitarne J, Sampietro GM, Serclova Z, Zmora O, Luglio G, de Buck van Overstraeten A, Burke JP, Buskens CJ, Colombo F, Dias JA, Eliakim R, Elosua T, Gecim IE, Kolacek S, Kierkus J, Kolho KL, Lefevre JH, Millan M, Panis Y, Pinkney T, Russell RK, Schwartz C, Vaizey C, Yassin N, D'Hoore A. ECCO-ESCP consensus on surgery for Crohn's disease. J Crohns Colitis. 2018;12:1–16.
9. Lightner AL, Jia X, Zaghiyan K, Fleshner PR. IPAA in known preoperative Crohn's disease: a systematic review. Dis Colon Rectum. 2021;64(3):355–64.
10. Pellino G, Vinci D, Signoriello G, Kontovounisios C, Canonico S, Selvaggi F, Sciaudone G. Long-term bowel function and fate of the ileal pouch after restorative proctocolectomy in patients with Crohn's disease: a systematic review with meta-analysis and metaregression. J Crohns Colitis. 2020;14(3):418–27.
11. Challine A, Voron T, O'Connell L, Chafai N, Debove C, Collard M, Parc Y, Lefèvre JH. Does an ileo-anal anastomosis decrease the rate of successful pregnancy compared to an ileorectal anastomosis? A national study of 1,491 patients. Ann Surg. 2023;277:806–12. https://doi.org/10.1097/SLA.0000000000005569.
12. Lee S, Crowe M, Seow CH, Kotze PG, Kaplan GG, Metcalfe A, et al. Surgery for inflammatory bowel disease has unclear impact on female fertility: a Cochrane collaboration systematic review. J Can Soc Gastroenterol. 2020;4(3):115–24.
13. Rottoli M, Pezzuto P, Fallani G, Pellino G, Rizzello F, Gionchetti P, et al. Ileal pouch-anal anastomosis in women of childbearing age affected by ulcerative colitis: a single-center study on the risk factors for infertility and outcomes of pregnancy over 17 years. J Crohns Colitis. 2022;16(Suppl 1):i259–61.
14. Goto Y, Uchino M, Horio Y, Kusunoki K, Minagawa T, Kuwahara R, et al. Delivery mode after ileal pouch-anal anastomosis among pregnant women with ulcerative colitis. J Anus Rectum Colon. 2021;5(4):419–25.
15. Park J, Gessler B, Block M, Angenete E. Complications and morbidity associated with loop ileostomies in patients with ulcerative colitis. Scand J Surg. 2018;107(1):38–42.
16. Khan F, Shen B. Complications related to J-pouch surgery. Gastroenterol Hepatol (N Y). 2018;14(10):571–6.
17. Deputy M, Segal J, Reza L, Worley G, Costello S, Burns E, et al. The pouch behaving badly: management of morbidity after ileal pouch–anal anastomosis. Color Dis. 2021;23:1193–204.

Chapter 8
Transanal Endoscopic Microsurgery

Emeka Ray-Offor

Introduction

Endoscopic therapies and local excision of benign and early malignant rectal tumors are attractive alternatives to more invasive surgeries. Generally, endoscopic techniques are favored in the setting of benign/ early cT1N0 rectal neoplasms given their decreased morbidity and increased cost-effectiveness [1]. Simple endoscopic therapies such as loop polypectomy and advanced techniques of endoscopic mucosal resection (EMR) may be inadequate for en bloc resection of larger size adenoma with a piecemeal endoscopic removal. Endoscopic mucosal dissection (ESD) facilitates a wider but non-full-thickness local rectal wall excision unlike the traditional Park's transanal excision (TAE) [2]. TAE involves the use of self-retaining rectal retraction under direct monocular vision facilitating a full-thickness local excision [3]. This direct access to a rectal lesion by TAE spares the morbidities associated with intra-abdominal approaches. However, this is limited by inadequate visualization of mid and upper rectal lesions hence the quest for more effective options.

Transanal endoscopic microsurgery (TEM) is an advancement of local excision techniques for rectal lesions introduced by Gerhard Buess et al. in 1984 [4, 5]. The equipment for this, manufactured by Richard Wolf (Knittlingen, Germany), utilizes a 40-mm diameter binocular operating endoscope coupled to the OR table by a rigid platform for operation using long in-line instruments with an insufflating system (Fig. 8.1). Saclaride et al. in 1998 published the first reported cases series in the

E. Ray-Offor (✉)
College of Health Sciences, University of Port Harcourt, Choba, Rivers State, Nigeria

Colorectal/Minimal Access Surgery Unit, Department of Surgery, University of Port Harcourt Teaching Hospital, Port Harcourt, Rivers State, Nigeria

Digestive Disease Unit, Oak Endoscopy Centre, Port Harcourt, Rivers State, Nigeria
e-mail: emeka.ray-offor@uniport.edu.ng

Fig. 8.1 (**a** and **b**) TEM platform and insufflation pump, respectively (Richard Wolf, Knittlingen, Germany)

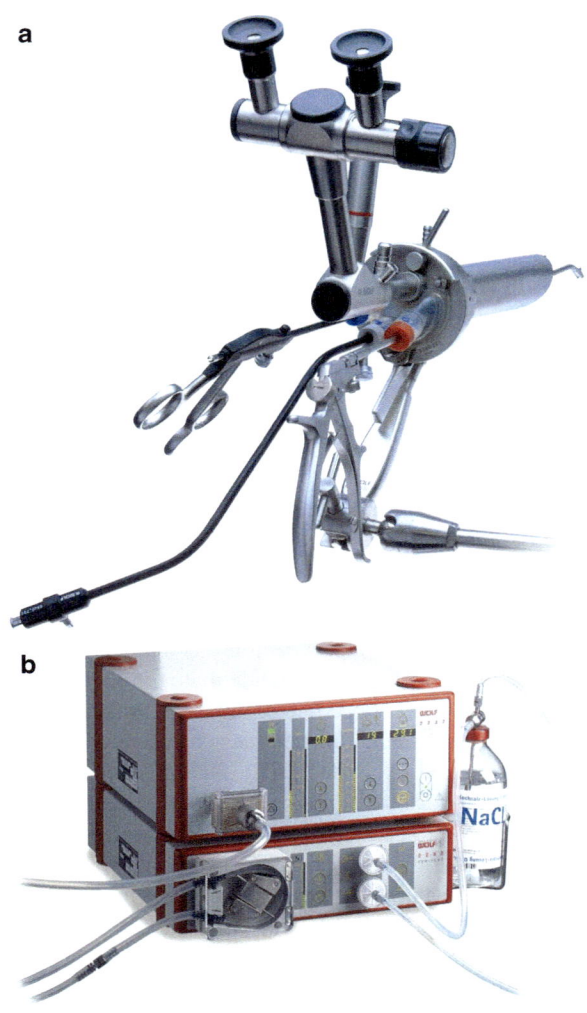

United States [6]. Ever since numerous studies have highlighted the utility of TEM in the treatment of adenomas and early rectal adenocarcinoma with a higher yield of negative margins [7–11]. TEM facilitates en-bloc resection of early rectal lesions by dissecting submucosally or by full-thickness rectal wall excision to the extent of the upper rectum in contrast to TAE. Despite these advantages, a wide application of this advanced transanal excision technique has been limited by a significant cost implication for the acquisition of the requisite equipment and a steep learning curve.

The resectoscope has been successfully combined with a two-dimensional panoramic view, conventional laparoscopic, and proprietary angled instruments in the TEO® platform (Karl Storz, Tuttlingen, Germany), to the familiarity of laparoscopic surgeons [12]. Further evolution has seen the successful transanal application of flexible single incision laparoscopic ports and its modification in the technique of transanal minimally invasive surgery TAMIS in contradistinction to rigid platforms of TEM and TEO [13]. Where expertise in these techniques exists the choice of platform to use is dependent on the surgeon's preference, availability, and cost [14, 15].

Indications

Giant Sessile Polyps

TEM as an advanced transanal excision technique is a suitable alternative for the treatment of giant sessile polyps. [16]

cT1N0

In line with the NCCN guideline, TEM is suitable for mobile, well to moderately differentiated, cT1N0 lesions that are less than 3 cm in diameter with no lymphovascular or perineural invasion within 8 cm and above 8 cm from the anal verge [17]. Lesions larger than 3 cm may also be eligible for local excision depending on the risk of postoperative rectal lumen stenosis.

cT2N0

TEM is a viable organ preservation option for en bloc resection in select T2 N0 rectal tumors located within 8 cm of the anal verge tumors following neoadjuvant chemoradiotherapy [18]. These patients are spared the possibility of permanent stoma, or urinary and sexual dysfunction that are associated with TME resection. The TREC trial showed that short-course radiotherapy and TEM were well tolerated in older and frailer patients, had good rates of organ preservation, and were associated with low rates of acute and long-term toxicity, with minimal effects on quality of life and functional status [19].

Palliative Resection

In addition, transanal surgery may present a palliative resection option for patients who are not candidates for diverting stomas either due to medical comorbidities or have failed diversion and are still experiencing pain or bleeding.

Contraindication

Patients presenting with suspected lymph nodal involvement or known T2–T3 cancer are usually not offered TEM.

Preoperative Preparation

Before surgery, a clinical evaluation of the patient is done involving a complete colonoscopy with biopsy and transanal ultrasonography. For rectal cancer patients, tumor staging involves magnetic resonance imaging and computed tomographic (CT) scans. In the consenting process for TEM, patients must be informed that a final pathological analysis may yield high-risk factors and necessitate additional radical surgery. Full-bowel mechanical preparation is administered the day before surgery with polyethylene glycol or sodium picosulphate magnesium citrate. Also, thromboembolic prophylaxis with low-molecular-weight heparin and a calf compression device is recommended.

The OR equipment is prechecked comprising the TEM platform and instruments.

TEO instrument comprises a 7, 15, or 20-cm rectal tube with a 40 mm diameter that has multiple channels for the introduction of dedicated or conventional laparoscopic instruments and a 5 mm optic telescope (Fig. 8.2) [20]. This platform incorporates a U-shaped holding system which is coupled to the OR table.

Anesthesia

General anesthesia with skeletal muscle relaxation is commonly used for TEM. Also, spinal anesthesia may be used when not contraindicated.

Fig. 8.2 TEO platform (© KARL STORZ SE & Co. KG, Germany)

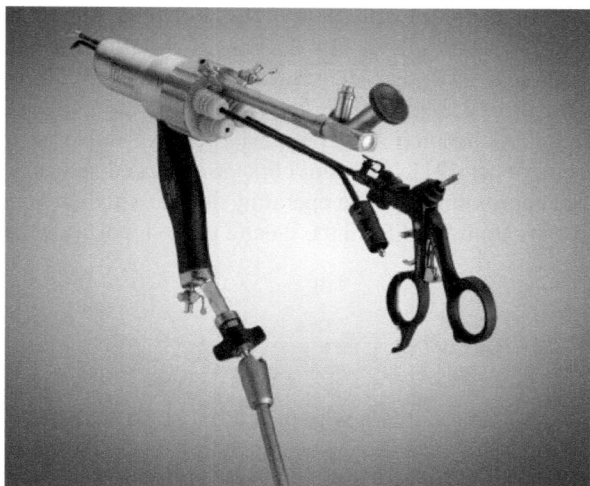

Positioning

The patient is positioned in a lithotomy or prone position depending on the tumor location to have the lesion as close as possible to the 6 o'clock position. The surgeon is seated to operate between the legs of the patient with the monitor positioned in front of him/her; the assistant is seated to the left of the surgeon. A Foley urethral catheter is inserted into the bladder before the start of surgery.

Technique

The abdomen, perineum, and thigh of the patient are prepped and draped in the usual sterile manner. The proctoscope is carefully inserted into the rectum and positioned by attaching it to the frame. Pneumorectum is created by the introduction of carbon dioxide to a pressure of 10–12 mmHg. Dissection is started at the inferior pole of the lesion using the monopolar electrode aiming for an adequate circumferential macroscopic clearance relative to the lesion. In full-thickness rectal wall excision, an ultrasonic energy device is preferable to prevent perforation. The specimen is retrieved transanal, pinned on a corkboard then sent to the pathology lab. Care is taken to identify peritoneal perforation and avoid injury to the urethra or vagina in females for anteriorly located rectal lesions.

The insufflation pressure of the pneumorectum is then reduced and closure of the defect is accomplished by interrupted 3-0 polydioxanone sutures secured by extracorporeal slipknots. The suturing of the rectal defect reduces the incidence of post-operative bleeding although it adds to operating time without significantly affecting length of hospital stay and post-operative infection in comparison to leaving the defect open [21]. Titanium clips or advanced suturing devices may be used for tissue approximation. The operating devices are then removed from the anal canal and patient transfered from the theatre to the recovery room in stable condition.

Post-operative Care

The urethral catheter is removed on #1 DPO. Patients are advised to resume diet 24–48 h after the operation, depending on the extent and type of resection, and usually are discharged after the first uneventful evacuation. A Gastrografin enema should be done before discharge if intraperitoneal entry takes place to ensure that there is no leak. Post-operative bleeding is a complication more common when the rectal defect is not sutured. Mucosal suturing can address this complication.

Special Notes

A valid alternative to non-disposable rigid trans-anal endoscopic microsurgery platforms is the use of disposable soft devices such as the Trans-anal Minimally Invasive Surgery (TAMIS). Based on the quality of local excision and perioperative complication both systems are equally effective although TAMIS resulted in less operative time consuming compared to TEM [22, 23]. The distal tip of the TEM system is typically beveled downward to facilitate operating on lesions in the dependent position. Patients must be positioned in lithotomy for posterior lesions, prone for anterior lesions, or in lateral decubitus for lateral lesions. Change in patient position can lengthen procedure time. The TAMIS ports are not beveled, and the increased working angle allows a 360-degree working space. Therefore, TAMIS can be completed in a lithotomy position regardless of the location of the lesion.

TEM can access more proximal lesions, has a specialized insufflator that permits a more stable pneumorectum, and has a significantly greater duration of patient follow-up in the surgical literature. TAMIS has a short learning curve, reduced device setup time, flexibility in instrument use, and application versatility. A cost-effective Insufflation tubing system and modern continuous flow systems have obviated the insufflation challenge of TAMIS. In terms of cost analysis TAMIS platform is cost-effective. Thie TEM platform has an initial capital cost of about US$80, 000, when compared to the TEO platform which costs approximately US$30,000.

Robotic transanal minimally invasive surgery (R-TAMIS) is an appealing alternative to transanal endoscopic microsurgery (TEM) and transanal minimally invasive surgery (TAMIS)) for benign and early malignant rectal lesions that are not amenable to traditional open transanal excision. It offers the oncologic benefits and perioperative complication profile of other transanal minimally invasive surgical approaches but also enhances surgeon ergonomics and provides an efficient transanal rectal platform [15, 24].

References

1. Naughton AP, Ryan ÉJ, Bardon CT, Boland MR, Aherne TM, Kelly ME, et al. Endoscopic management versus transanal surgery for early primary or early locally recurrent rectal neoplasms-a systematic review and meta-analysis. Int J Color Dis. 2020;35:2347–59.
2. Pimentel-Nunes P, Dinis-Ribeiro M, Ponchon T, Repici A, Vieth M, De Ceglie A, et al. Endoscopic submucosal dissection: European Society of Gastrointestinal Endoscopy (ESGE) guideline. Endoscopy. 2015;47:829–54.
3. Parks AG. A technique for excising extensive villous papillomatous change in the lower rectum. Proc R Soc Med. 1968;61(5):441–2.
4. Buess G, Hutterer F, Theiss J, Böbel M, Isselhard W, Pichlmaier H. A system for a transanal endoscopic rectum operation. Chirurg. 1984;55:677–80.
5. Buess G, Theiss R, Günther M, Hutterer F, Pichlmaier H. Endoscopic surgery in the rectum. Endoscopy. 1985;17:31–5.
6. Saclarides TJ. Transanal endoscopic microsurgery: a single surgeon's experience. Arch Surg. 1998;133(6):595–8; discussion 598–9.
7. Clancy C, Burke JP, Albert MR, O'Connell PR, Winter DC. Transanal endoscopic microsurgery versus standard transanal excision for the removal of rectal neoplasms: a systematic review and meta-analysis. Dis Colon Rectum. 2015;58:254–61.
8. Moore JS, Cataldo PA, Osler T, Hyman NH. Transanal endoscopic microsurgery is more effective than traditional transanal excision for resection of rectal masses. Dis Colon Rectum. 2008;51:1026–30; discussion 1030–1031.
9. Barendse RM, van den Broek FJ, Dekker E, Bemelman WA, de Graaf EJ, Fockens P, et al. Systematic review of endoscopic mucosal resection versus transanal endoscopic microsurgery for large rectal adenomas. Endoscopy. 2011;43:941–9.
10. de Graaf EJ, Burger JW, van Ijsseldijk AL, Tetteroo GW, Dawson I, Hop WC. Transanal endoscopic microsurgery is superior to transanal excision of rectal adenomas. Color Dis. 2011;13:762–7.
11. Lu JY, Lin GL, Qiu HZ, Xiao Y, Wu B, Zhou JL. Comparison of transanal endoscopic microsurgery and total mesorectal excision in the treatment of T1 rectal cancer: a meta-analysis. PLoS One. 2015;10(10):e0141427.
12. Nieuwenhuis DH, Draaisma WA, Verberne GH, van Overbeeke AJ, Consten EC. Transanal endoscopic operation for rectal lesions using two-dimensional visualization and standard endoscopic instruments: a prospective cohort study and comparison with the literature. Surg Endosc. 2009;23:80–6.
13. Mege D, Bridoux V, Maggiori L, Tuech JJ, Panis Y. What is the best tool for transanal endoscopic microsurgery (TEM)? A case-matched study in 74 patients comparing a standard platform and a disposable material. Int J Color Dis. 2017;32(7):1041–5.
14. Lee L, Edwards K, Hunter IA, Hartley JE, Atallah SB, Albert MR, et al. Quality of local excision for rectal neoplasms using transanal endoscopic microsurgery versus transanal minimally invasive surgery: a multi-institutional matched analysis. Dis Colon Rectum. 2017;60:928–35.
15. Emolo J, Ramos-Delgado D, Sands DR. When is transanal endoscopic surgery appropriate? Surg Oncol. 2022;43:101773.

16. Xiong X, Wang C, Wang B, Shen Z, Jiang K, Gao Z, et al. Can transanal endoscopic microsurgery effectively treat T1 or T2 rectal cancer? A systematic review and meta-analysis. Surg Oncol. 2021;37:101561.
17. Benson AB, Venook AP, Al-Hawary MM, Azad N, Chen YJ, Ciombor KK, et al. Rectal cancer, version 2.2022, NCCN clinical practice guidelines in oncology. J Natl Compr Cancer Netw. 2022;20(10):1139–67.
18. Gilbert A, Homer V, Brock K, Korsgen S, Geh I, Hill J, et al; TREC collaborators. Quality-of-life outcomes in older patients with early-stage rectal cancer receiving organ-preserving treatment with hypofractionated short-course radiotherapy followed by transanal endoscopic microsurgery (TREC): non-randomised registry of patients unsuitable for total mesorectal excision. Lancet Healthy Longev. 2022;3(12):e825-e838.
19. Morino M, Allaix ME. Transanal endoscopic microsurgery. In: Jaap Bonjer H, editor. Surgical principles of minimally invasive procedures. Springer.
20. Khan K, Hunter IA, Manzoor T. Should the rectal defect be sutured following TEMS/TAMIS carried out for neoplastic rectal lesions? A meta-analysis. An R Coll Surg Engl. 2020;102(9):647–53.
21. Stipa F, Tierno SM, Russo G, Burza A. Trans-anal minimally invasive surgery (TAMIS) versus trans-anal endoscopic microsurgery (TEM): a comparative case-control matched-pairs analysis. Surg Endosc. 2022;36(3):2081–6.
22. Perivoliotis K, Baloyiannis I, Sarakatsianou C, Tzovaras G. Comparison of the transanal surgical techniques for local excision of rectal tumors: a network meta-analysis. Int J Color Dis. 2020;35:1173–82.
23. Burke JP, Albert M. Transanal minimally invasive surgery (TAMIS): pros and cons of this evolving procedure. Semin Colon Rectal Surg. 2015;26(1):36–40.
24. Tomassi MJ, Taller J, Yuhan R, et al. Robotic transanal minimally invasive surgery for the excision of rectal neoplasia: clinical experience with 58 consecutive patients. Dis Colon Rectum. 2019;62(3):279–85.

Chapter 9
Transanal Minimally Invasive Surgery TAMIS

Matthew Albert and Paul M. Kaminsky

Introduction

The treatment of rectal neoplasms has evolved greatly over the last four decades. In addition to an aging population, the increasing implementation of screening programs worldwide, as well as improvements in radiologic evaluation, have led to an increasing incidence of early rectal neoplasm amenable to local excision. More importantly, surgical techniques and transanal access platforms, initially TEM (Transanal Endoscopic Microsurgery) and subsequently TAMIS (Transanal Minimally Invasive Surgery), have evolved to permit high-quality resection of rectal tumors. Compared to traditional local excision utilizing rectal retractors, both TEM and TAMIS have consistently and unequivocally demonstrated improved outcomes with decreased margin positivity, less tumor fragmentation, lower local recurrence rates, and higher long-term survival [1–3]. Conversely, radical resection (Low anterior resection and abdominoperineal resection) has excellent oncologic outcomes but is associated with significant morbidity and mortality, including anastomotic leak (5–15%), septic complications, sexual and bladder dysfunction, and permanent stoma [4]. The treatment of malignant neoplasms is a balance between the morbidity of classical radical surgery with the increased risk of recurrence with local excision.

Since the introduction of TAMIS in 2010, which utilized a single-incision laparoscopic surgery port, flexible access devices specifically FDA-approved for transanal surgery have been designed and are commercially available. (Gelpoint Path, Applied Medical, Rancho Santa Margarita) [5]. Widespread availability, shorter learning curve, and easy training and implementation have led to extensive adoption of TAMIS compared to other modalities in the last decade [6]. TAMIS is a valuable

---

M. Albert (✉) · P. M. Kaminsky
Advent Health Medical Group, Center for Colon and Rectal Surgery, Orlando, FL, USA
e-mail: Matthew.Albert.MD@adventhealth.com

© The Author(s), under exclusive license to Springer Nature Switzerland AG 2024
E. Ray-Offor, R. J. Rosenthal (eds.), *Colorectal & Hernia Laparoscopic Surgery*, https://doi.org/10.1007/978-3-031-63490-1_9

technique for local excision of lesions in the rectum that can be performed using readily available equipment and minimally invasive skills [7, 8].

Patient Selection

As cure rates for early rectal cancer are very high with radical surgery, local excision must offer cure rates comparable to radical surgery while allowing for improved functional outcomes and reduced morbidity. The main disadvantage of local excision compared to radical surgery is the inability to properly assess for lymph node metastases, and every effort must be made to select patients with minimal risk of lymph node involvement for curative local excision [9]. Published rates of lymph node metastasis (LNM) for all T1 and T2 rectal tumors range from 10–14% for T1 and ~20–25% for T2 [10–14]. However, when lesions with unfavorable pathology are excluded (poor differentiation, lymphovascular, and perineural invasion), these rates drop significantly (T1 2.2–6%, T2 11%) [10, 12]. The National Comprehensive Cancer Network rectal cancer guidelines state that patients with mobile, well to moderately differentiated, cT1N0 lesions that are less than 3 cm in diameter with no lymphovascular or perineural invasion are appropriate candidates for local excision. Lesions larger than 3 cm may also be eligible for local excision depending on the risk of postoperative rectal lumen stenosis. Although current recommendations suggest that lesions that demonstrate invasion deeper than the first third of the submucosa (i.e. sm2/3) are at higher risk of lymph node metastases, recent literature suggests that sm2 tumors with favorable pathology have rates of LNM similar to sm1 [10–12, 14].

Strict adherence to these criteria may result in equivalent oncologic outcomes for local excision compared to radical surgery. An analysis of the Surveillance, Epidemiology, and End Results database reported that comparable cancer-specific survival between local excision and transabdominal resection [15], and a meta-analysis comparing TEM local excision and radical surgery for T1 rectal cancer also demonstrated equivalent 5-year overall survival [3, 16]. Additionally, patients must be informed that a final pathological analysis may yield high-risk factors and warrant additional radical surgery.

Patients with T1 sm3 or T2 tumors who are considered high-risk for radical surgery or patients with tumors that would result in a permanent stoma may consider local excision, albeit with informed discussion over the increased risk of local and mesorectal recurrence (OR 2 of lymph node metastasis in T1 vs. T2 tumors), in the context of current guidelines and patient desired outcomes [10, 11]. Treatment of these tumors should be discussed in a multidisciplinary setting, particularly regarding any benefit of adjuvant chemoradiation therapy.

Patients with T3 tumors with a response to neoadjuvant therapy are also being considered for local excision, however, the authors caution that a complete pathologic response in the primary tumor does not imply a complete nodal response. T3 tumors frequently have nodal metastasis (40–50%) and may have positive nodes despite a complete pathologic response in the primary tumor [10, 17]. Therefore, we do not recommend local excision in these cases unless the patient cannot tolerate radical surgery.

There are no specific contraindications for TAMIS local excision other than those outlined above. Lesions that are located within 3 cm of the anal verge may be difficult to fully access by TAMIS due to the length of the operating port (37–44 mm in length), which may obscure the distal extent of the lesion. This concern is not limited to TAMIS, as the TEM rectoscope also presents important difficulties in obtaining a proper seal for very distal lesions. For these cases, a hybrid approach in which dissection of the distal-most aspect is begun transanal, then the TAMIS port is introduced to finish the proximal dissection. This approach allows for the advantages of the advanced endoscopic platforms to be applied for lesions that would otherwise be at high risk of R1 resection and fragmentation by traditional TAE.

Preoperative Evaluation

Preoperative evaluation begins with a detailed history, including disease-specific and associated symptoms, family history, as well as performance status, functional capacity to undergo surgery, and physical examination with attention to digital rectal examination. Lesions that can be palpated by digital rectal exam should be assessed as to whether they are firm, mobile, or fixed in addition to the exact location of the anorectal ring. Full endoscopic evaluation of the colon must be performed to rule out synchronous lesions that may change the management strategy. This must be combined with rigid proctosigmoidoscopy by the operating surgeon to assess tumor size, location within the lumen, distance of the lower and upper extent of the tumor from the anal verge, and circumferential extent. Care should also be taken to document preoperative sphincter function by history, physical examination, and patient-reported fecal incontinence scores if needed.

Local staging of the tumor must also be performed. Depending on local availability and expertise, transrectal ultrasound (TRUS) and pelvic magnetic resonance imaging (MRI) may be used as a sole modality or in combination. Older studies have demonstrated the superiority of TRUS over MRI for depth of invasion assessment, while MRI may be superior to determining lymph node involvement [18]. However, there is increasing data supporting the superiority of MRI over TRUS in identifying favorable lesions for local excision, and is currently recommended by the National Accreditation Program for Rectal Cancer [19–21]. At our institution, all patients undergo three Tesla MRIs for local staging. Computed tomography of the chest, abdomen, and pelvis and carcinoembryonic antigen level to rule out distant metastasis completes the staging evaluation. Routine laboratory investigations and positron emission tomography (PET) scans are not necessary and increase costs without altering management decisions. Once the preoperative evaluation is complete, patients should be presented at a multidisciplinary tumor board to arrive at a consensus management plan. Interestingly, for pathologically and clinically benign villous lesions, we intentionally omit further radiologic evaluation in favor of full-thickness excisional biopsy, as overstating and potentially overtreatment are quite common.

Technical Aspects/Operative Technique

Mechanical bowel preparation is essential in TAMIS as a clear operative field is required to operate endoluminal. A simple enema preparation is often sufficient. In the setting of poor preparation, high-volume irrigation utilizing a rigid proctoscope can easily be performed. Patients with mid-rectal anterior lesions should all undergo complete preparation to minimize contamination in case of peritoneal entry. Current evidence supports the use of oral antibiotics in addition to a mechanical bowel preparation in patients undergoing a large bowel anastomosis for a reduction in wound-related complications, however, its effect in transanal surgery is unclear.

Surgical site infection and thromboprophylaxis are given within 30 min of surgery according to guidelines for colonic surgery. Foley catheterization is optional as urinary retention is rare.

Patients can be placed in a lithotomy position regardless of lesion position within the rectal lumen. The main operative monitor is placed at the head of the operative bed and both surgeon and assistant are seated between the legs of the patient. Basic laparoscopic instruments (including graspers, monopolar cautery, and needle drivers) can be used. A 5 mm angled (30–45 °) scope is preferable as it offsets the operating surgeon's hands and minimizes instrument collision as well as displaying a more circumferential view of the rectum compared to a nonangled camera. An angled camera also facilitates assessment of the lateral and proximal margins and can improve visualization around the rectal valves. Simple monopolar cautery, as well as energy devices, can all be utilized for dissection and hemostasis. Monopolar cautery is preferable, providing greater precision and is more cost-effective. A suction device is most commonly used to facilitate smoke evacuation, in addition to controlling minor bleeding or removal of fecal contents. Combined suction and monopolar devices designed for TAMIS are highly beneficial in providing both functions.

Following a perianal block and dilatation of the anal canal, the access port is inserted and secured, and the gel cap, which contains the trocars is placed. Pneumorectum is created with carbon dioxide insufflation kept at 15-18 mmHg and can be increased up to 20 mm Hg if required. Newer generation insufflators (AirSeal Insufflation System, ConMed, Inc. Denver, CO) and Stryker Pneumosure with TAMIS mode (Stryker Endoscopy, Kalamazoo, MI)have dramatically improved the stability of pneomorectum. The development of an Insufflation Stabilization Bag (ISB) used in conjunction with the Gelpoint Path, provides a cost-effective alternative to newer insufflators. Traditional laparoscopic instruments are then introduced through the gelport for dissection.

A complete assessment of the tumor is performed with any bleeding from port insertion trauma gently irrigated. Precise extension of the lesion, especially in large carpeting adenomas, is easily assessed with a high-definition laparoscope. A quality excision, defined as a non-fragmented, full-thickness, margin-negative tumor resection is mandatory for the treatment of early rectal cancer by local excision no matter the technique used. The procedure begins with the marking out of the lesion with at least a 1 cm margin circumferentially using electrocautery (Fig. 9.1a and b). Full-thickness division of the rectal wall distal to the lesion is then performed, which allows manipulation of the specimen without direct contact with the tumor. Perpendicular division through the entire rectal wall until the mesorectal fat is encountered is critical to achieving a complete specimen (Fig. 9.2a and b). During excision and manipulation, the specimen must be grasped on the edge of normal mucosa or underneath the lesion on the mesorectal fat to minimize fragmentation of the tissue and tumor. Although controversial, some surgeons advocate en bloc removal of mesorectal fat beneath the lesion to retrieve lymph nodes, especially when the lesion is located posteriorly in the rectum. No literature supporting the superiority of this technique exists, though theoretically the sampling of positive or negative lymph nodes potentially may significantly alter treatment recommendations. This notion is supported by several small studies of sentinel lymph node

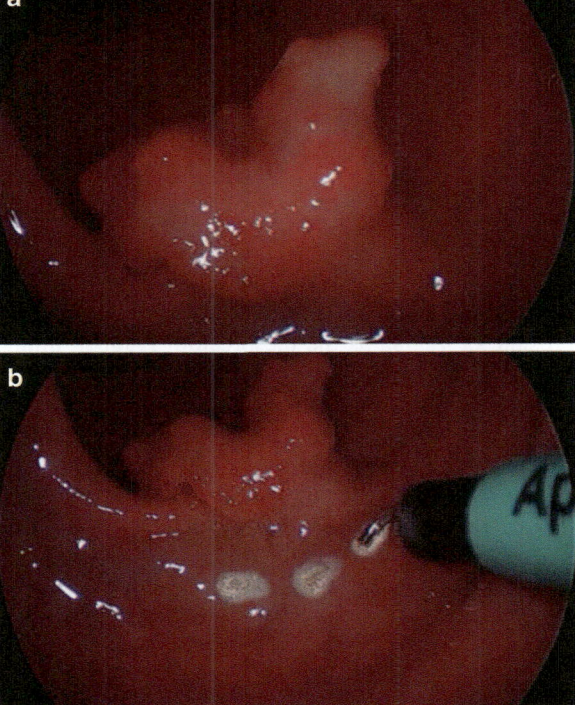

Fig. 9.1 (a and b) Lesion being marked out during TAMIS local excision. A monopolar cautery device is used to score the rectal mucosa with a 1 cm circumferential margin

Fig. 9.2 (**a** and **b**) Full-thickness excision. Note the mesorectal fat underneath the lesion, signifying that the entire rectal wall has been transected

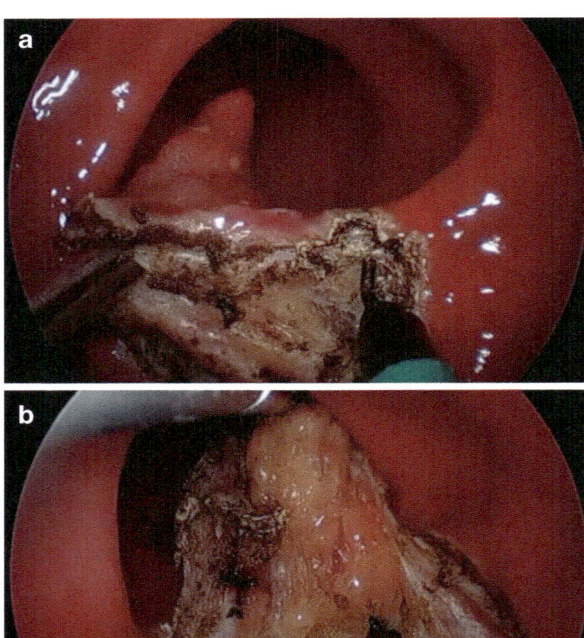

biopsy in rectal cancer. The dye-containing nodes are typically near the primary tumor. Care must be taken to avoid breaching the mesorectal fascial envelope to minimize disruption of the anatomic planes should proctectomy become necessary [8].

Anterior lesions are still best accessed in the lithotomy position, in contrast to conventional transanal excision or TEM where the prone jackknife position is necessary. Particular attention must be paid to anterior lesions to avoid injury to the prostate or vagina as the mesorectum is much thinner. Anterior organ injury was described in the early literature of TEM in the 1980's, however, has not been reported in any series on TAMIS. Familiarity with the anatomical planes and surrounding critical structures is important. Peritoneal entry is an uncommon event, occurring in up to 4% of patients with anterior tumors located in the mid and upper rectum. If this occurs, mandatory closure of the rectal wall is performed by first closing the peritoneum and then the rectal wall. Transient loss of pneumorectum may occur but is re-established following peritoneal closure. Rarely, laparoscopic access is required to cleanse the pelvis, facilitate wall closure, or perform a leak test. Informed consent in patients at risk of peritoneal entry should be performed.

Following resection, the specimen should be immediately retrieved and oriented. It should be pinned out and sent to the pathologist as a fresh, non-preserved specimen to facilitate margin evaluation. A positive margin for rectal cancer should be re-excised or converted to formal radical surgery.

Following removal, it is our practice to irrigate the defect with betadine to minimize bacteria and tumor contamination (Fig. 9.3). It is the practice of our institution to then close full-thickness defects transversely with interrupted or continuous suturing to avoid narrowing the lumen (Fig. 9.4). The pneomorectum is decreased to 7–8 mmHg to reduce tension on the suture lines. A running closure beginning in the lateral portion of the incision can be achieved but is technically more challenging. The use of a V-Loc™ suture (Covidien, Mansfield, MA) can expedite continuous closure by maintaining tension and negating the need for knot-tying. Conversely, closure can be performed in an interrupted fashion with knot tying facilitated by laparoscopic knot pushers. Alternatively, the defect can be left to heal with the expectation of a minimal scar within 4–6 weeks and few complications. Hahnloser et al. reported outcomes from 75 TAMIS excisions performed at three centers and found no difference in complications between closed defects and those that were left open [22]. A rigid or flexible sigmoidoscopy can be done at the end of the procedure so access the luminal diameter if there are any concerns.

TAMIS is a treatment option following neoadjuvant chemoradiotherapy although this continues to be evaluated in clinical trials. However, despite multiple different closure techniques described, wound dehiscence in this setting, with accompanying pain, hospital admission, and the occasional need for fecal diversion is common [8].

TAMIS has been performed robotically with success [23, 24]. However, robot docking time, which can be up to 36 min [24], as well as the additional costs incurred by the use of the robot equipment (up to 1000 Euro per patient, excluding capital expenditure on the robot system and its maintenance) limits the applicability of robotic TAMIS.

Fig. 9.3 Irrigated defect

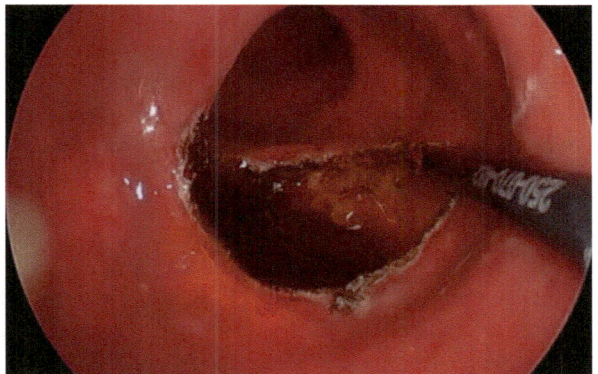

Fig. 9.4 Rectal wall defect closure

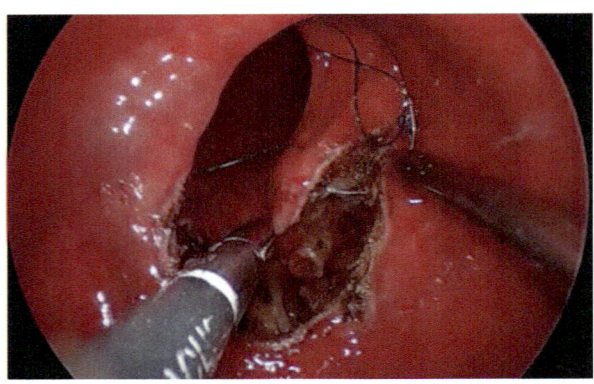

Post-operative Care

TAMIS is feasible to perform on an outpatient basis. In patients with advanced age, significant comorbidities, or an increased risk of bleeding, selective overnight admission can be considered. In our experience of over 350 patients, nearly 80% underwent same-day discharge. All patients must be counseled on the signs of early and late postoperative hemorrhage and pelvic sepsis. In addition, transient rectal discharge and short-term changes in bowel habits are expected. A regular diet is initiated once recovered from anesthesia. Opioids, non-steroidal anti-inflammatories, or acetaminophen can be prescribed orally at discharge depending on pain levels. Narcotics are frequently unnecessary, except in tumors where the incision or closure abuts the dentate line. Postoperative antibiotics are not recommended.

A postoperative evaluation of the patient within a multidisciplinary team is a mandatory component of performing TAMIS for rectal cancer. A complete pathologic review, including depth of submucosal invasion as well as high-risk features, is critical for appropriate decision-making. Tumors with final pathology demonstrating poor histological features or a tumor stage T1 sm3 or greater should be evaluated for total mesorectal excision. Patients with T2 tumors who underwent local excision have increased rates of local recurrence and shorter overall survival compared to radical surgery, but this difference was not present in patients with T2 tumors who underwent neoadjuvant therapy [25]. The TESAR trial (NCT02371304) will further examine the oncologic outcomes of patients with T1–2 tumors who undergo neoadjuvant therapy and local excision vs. radical surgery alone [26]. However, it is reasonable to consider adjuvant therapy for a patient who underwent local resection with T2 final pathology and who cannot undergo radical surgery [27]. There is no consensus about the timing of radical surgery and the role of adjuvant medical treatment in this setting, however, delay of surgery to permit healing over 4–6 weeks is usual to minimize inflammatory disruption of surgical planes. Data from patients undergoing TEM and followed by radical resection does show a reduction in the quality of the TME performed when compared to similar patients treated by TME alone [28]. However, initial studies of salvage TME through a transanal approach have improved the pathologic quality of TME specimens [29].

Complications

As with traditional TAE and TEM, local excision utilizing TAMIS has a low complication rate with low severity, especially when compared to radical surgery. However, knowledge of the risk factors, diagnosis, and management of this unique set of complications is critical for any surgeon performing TAMIS.

Bleeding is the most common complication associated with TAMIS and is usually self-limited. Bleeding can occur early after surgery or be delayed in presentation often related to suture line dehiscence. In our experience, most postoperative bleeding can be successfully managed without further intervention. Patients who fail conservative management may require endoscopic evaluation with injection or coagulation, or examination under anesthesia with over-sewing of the offending vessel.

The incidence of wound dehiscence following TAMIS is unclear, as symptoms are self-limited. Examination after 30 days nearly always demonstrates complete healing regardless of whether the defect was closed or not. However, suture line dehiscence after peritoneal entry has the obvious potential to lead to more significant complications such as pelvic sepsis. More importantly, local excision following neoadjuvant therapy is associated with a high incidence of wound breakdown, severe pain, and readmission, and may even require fecal diversion. In a series by Marks et al., morbidity following patients who underwent neoadjuvant chemoradiation followed by TEM, a 25.6% wound complication rate was reported with one patient requiring diversion [30]. Perez et al. reported suture line dehiscence rates of 60.9% with 43.5% of patients requiring readmission, and have since abandoned this approach [31]. In a smaller subset of patients, our experience has mirrored those described above, with one patient developing sepsis with an extra sphincteric fistula. Nonetheless, this approach continues to generate interest in the quest for organ-preserving therapy.

Fever has been reported following TAMIS, which may be caused by transient bacteremia. Observation is generally safe, and antibiotics are usually not necessary. However, the persistence of high fever and other signs of a systemic inflammatory response requires further evaluation. As with most any anorectal operation, urinary retention requiring catheterization has been reported with TAMIS but is uncommon (2%) [32]. The incidence of urinary retention after TEM has been reported to be as high as 8% and is hypothesized to be secondary to compression of the anterior rectal wall and urethra with the endoscope. Minimal pressure is applied to these structures in TAMIS as the port is softer and deploys below the level of the prostate. Resolution following catheterization should be expected. More serious urologic complications such as rectourethral fistula have not been reported with TAMIS but could result from any urethral injury following deep dissection of an anterior lesion. In our series, one patient developed scrotal emphysema/pneumoscrotum without peritoneal entry, which resolved spontaneously.

Transient fecal incontinence may occur following TAMIS. Anal dilatation from the 4 cm access channel is probably the biggest contributor and is likely to be related to the duration of surgery. Loss of rectal volume and compliance, due to the reduction of rectum following partial removal, in addition to increased mucous production in the healing rectum are likely additional causative factors. As with TEM, incontinence is generally temporary with restoration of normal function and manometric parameters at 6 months. Karakayli et al. evaluated anorectal function after TAMIS for rectal tumors in 10 patients and found no difference in preoperative and postoperative anorectal manometry at 3 weeks [33]. Only mean minimal sensory volumes were lower after surgery. Cleveland Clinic Incontinence Scores were also normal in all patients at 6 weeks. Similarly, Verseveld et al. reported no detrimental impact of TAMIS on quality of life or anorectal function in 24 patients undergoing TAMIS [34].

Peritoneal entry following full-thickness excision of anterior tumors has occurred with TAMIS, in 1–4% of patients, similar to TEM [35]. Given the locations of the peritoneal reflection in men and women, surgeons should be prepared to encounter this challenge when operating on any lesion anteriorly in the mid-rectum. In one study, by multivariate analysis, tumor distance ≥7 cm from the anal verge was the only independent predictor for peritoneal entry [36]. The risk of pelvic infection or tumor recurrence has not been demonstrated with increased incidence in most reports.

Knowledge of the treatment and morbidity after peritoneal violation has largely evolved from TEM experience over the last 30 years. In the infancy of TEM, peritoneal perforation frequently required conversion to laparotomy, resection, and creation of permanent or protective stomas. This has since evolved to the current management of peritoneal entry, which can be closed in two layers of the peritoneum and the full-thickness rectal wall. Alternatively, conversion to laparoscopy or laparotomy with transabdominal wall closure and leak test can be performed with or without a protective stoma. Not surprisingly, the learning curve and case volume seem to influence the treatment strategy employed when this occurs. In series of less than 100 patients, transabdominal access is obtained for 50–100% of the cases of peritoneal entry, whereas this incidence decreases to 0–40% in series larger than 100 patients. Salm et al. reported that conversion rates to laparotomy significantly decreased with experience, from 11.6% of surgeons with less than 10 TEM procedures to 1.2% of surgeons with more than 100 procedures [37]. Peritoneal entry seems not to be associated with any higher risk of pelvic infection. Given these data, simple endoluminal closure is likely adequate. In our experience of more than 350 TAMIS procedures, conversion to transabdominal laparoscopic closure occurred more frequently within our first 100 procedures but was more likely associated with the use of a traditional laparoscopic insufflator which often failed to maintain stable pneumorectum to permit safe endoluminal closure.

Long-term oncological safety has also been a primary concern associated with peritoneal entry, especially when operating on malignant lesions. Initial concerns of tumor seeding the peritoneum after transrectal perforation have been unfounded as multiple high-volume series have not supported any increased risk of recurrence or metastasis. Nonetheless, this risk can potentially be avoided in the early experience of TAMIS by careful patient selection.

Follow Up

Close clinical and endoscopic follow-up is vital to the detection of local and systemic recurrence. By the National Comprehensive Cancer Network (NCCN) guidelines, patients should undergo a history, physical examination, rigid proctoscopy, and serum CEA level every 3 months for 2 years, then every 6 months for a total of 5 years after excision of a malignant lesion. A full colonoscopy at 1- and 3-years following resection should be performed and every 5 years thereafter to identify metachronous lesions. It is the authors' practice to supplement the radiologic evaluation with a pelvic MRI to identify suspicious lymph nodes every 6 months for the first 2 years following resection.

Outcome/Current Results

Since its introduction in 2009, there have been over 550 published TAMIS cases for local excision of rectal neoplasia [22, 32, 38, 39]. Perioperative outcomes are excellent as morbidity and mortality after TAMIS is low—the overall complication rate was 7.4% in a systematic review of 390 TAMIS cases and there were no mortalities. There also does not appear to be any impairment in anorectal function or quality of life after TAMIS [34, 40]. Resection quality in experienced hands is also well in line with TEM data. In our own experience of 200 procedures for local excision of rectal neoplasia of which 55% were performed for malignancy, 93% of patients had an R0 resection and 95% of patients had an en bloc resection. Overall, 6% of patients experienced a local recurrence after a mean follow-up period in our institutional cohort of 14.4 months but was only 1% in patients with invasive disease and in whom TAMIS was performed with curative intent. Keller et al. reported similar results in their series of 75 cases, with a margin positivity rate of 6.6% and less than 1% tumor fragmentation rate [38]. They reported a local recurrence rate of 5.8% after a mean follow-up of 36.5 months [41]. These data compare favorably with traditional TAE, as TEM is associated with significantly lower margin positivity, tumor fragmentation, and local recurrence rates [2]. There were also no differences in 5-year overall or disease-specific survival between radical surgery and TEM for early rectal cancer, but TEM was associated with a higher risk of local recurrence [3]. However, TEM was associated with significantly lower perioperative morbidity and mortality compared to radical surgery. There are no data specifically comparing TAMIS and radical surgery, and thus much of the data are extrapolated from TEM. TAMIS is a versatile platform that offers colorectal surgeons a much broader application than for local excision of rectal neoplasia. This ability to approach diseases of the rectum with a different perspective has applications in the repair of a recto-urethral fistula, foreign body retrieval, ligation of rectal Dieulafoy lesion, completion proctectomy, and trans-anal total mesorectal excision (taTME) [42]. TAMIS beyond local excision is likely to expand as surgeons become more experienced with this emerging technique [43–49].

References

1. Morson BC, Bussey HJ, Samoorian S. Policy of local excision for early cancer of the colorectum. Gut. 1977;18:1045–50.
2. Clancy C, Burke JP, Albert MR, O'Connell PR. Winter DC Transanal endoscopic microsurgery versus standard transanal excision for the removal of rectal neoplasms: a systematic review and meta-analysis. Dis Colon Rectum. 2015;58:254–61.
3. Kidane B, Chadi SA, Kanters S, Colquhoun PH, Ott MC. Local resection compared with radical resection in the treatment of T1N0M0 rectal adenocarcinoma: a systematic review and meta-analysis. Dis Colon Rectum. 2015;58:122–40.
4. Lu ZR, Rajendran N, Lynch AC, Heriot AG, Warrier SK. Anastomotic leaks after restorative resections for rectal cancer compromise cancer outcomes and survival. Dis Colon Rectum. 2016;59:236–44.
5. Buess G, Hutterer F, Theiss J, Bobel M, Isselhard W, et al. A system for a transanal endoscopic rectum operation. Chirurg. 1984;55:677–80.
6. Winde G, Nottberg H, Keller R, Schmid KW, Bunte H. Surgical cure for early rectal carcinomas (T1). Transanal endoscopic microsurgery vs. anterior resection. Dis Colon Rectum. 1996;39:969–76.
7. Atallah S, Albert M, Larach S. Transanal minimally invasive surgery: a giant leap forward. Surg Endosc. 2010;24:2200–5.
8. deBeche-Adams T, Nassif G. Transanal minimally invasive surgery. Clin Colon Rectal Surg. 2015;28:176–80.
9. Glasgow SC, Bleier JI, Burgart LJ, Finne CO, Lowry AC. Meta-analysis of histopathological features of primary colorectal cancers that predict lymph node metastases. J Gastrointest Surg. 2012;16:1019–28.
10. Saraste D, Gunnarsson U, Janson M. Predicting lymph node metastases in early rectal cancer. Eur J Cancer. 2013;49:1104–8.
11. Han J, Hur H, Min BS, Lee KY, Kim NK. Predictive factors for lymph node metastasis in submucosal invasive colorectal carcinoma: a new proposal of depth of invasion for radical surgery. World J Surg. 2018;42:2635–41.
12. Oka S, Tanaka S, Nakadoi K, Kanao H, Chayama K. Risk analysis of submucosal invasive rectal carcinomas for lymph node metastasis to expand indication criteria for endoscopic resection. Dig Endosc. 2013;25 Suppl 2:21–5.
13. Okabe S, Shia J, Nash G, Wong WD, Guillem JG, et al. Lymph node metastasis in T1 adenocarcinoma of the colon and rectum. J Gastrointest Surg. 2004;8:1032–9. discussion 1039–1040
14. Nascimbeni R, Burgart LJ, Nivatvongs S, Larson DR. Risk of lymph node metastasis in T1 carcinoma of the colon and rectum. Dis Colon Rectum. 2002;45:200–6.
15. Bhangu A, Brown G, Nicholls RJ, Wong J, Darzi A, et al. Survival outcome of local excision versus radical resection of colon or rectal carcinoma: a surveillance, epidemiology, and end results (SEER) population-based study. Ann Surg. 2013;258:563–9; discussion 569–571

16. Lu JY, Lin GL, Qiu HZ, Xiao Y, Wu B, et al. Comparison of transanal endoscopic microsurgery and total mesorectal excision in the treatment of T1 rectal cancer: a meta-analysis. PLoS One. 2015;10:e0141427.
17. Tranchart H, Lefevre JH, Svrcek M, Flejou JF, Tiret E, et al. What is the incidence of metastatic lymph node involvement after a significant pathologic response of primary tumor following neoadjuvant treatment for locally advanced rectal cancer? Ann Surg Oncol. 2013;20:1551–9.
18. Bipat S, Glas AS, Slors FJ, Zwinderman AH, Bossuyt PM, et al. Rectal cancer: local staging and assessment of lymph node involvement with endoluminal US, CT, and MR imaging—a meta-analysis. Radiology. 2004;232:773–83.
19. An C, Huh H, Han KH, Kim MJ, Kim NK, et al. Use of preoperative MRI to select candidates for local excision of MRI-staged T1 and T2 rectal cancer: can MRI select patients with N0 tumors? Dis Colon Rectum. 2015;58:923–30.
20. Mondal D, Betts M, Cunningham C, Mortensen NJ, Lindsey I, et al. How useful is endorectal ultrasound in the management of early rectal carcinoma? Int J Color Dis. 2014;29:1101–4.
21. Brown G, Davies S, Williams GT, Bourne MW, Newcombe RG, et al. Effectiveness of preoperative staging in rectal cancer: digital rectal examination, endoluminal ultrasound, or magnetic resonance imaging? Br J Cancer. 2004;91:23–9.
22. Hahnloser D, Cantero R, Salgado G, Dindo D, Rega D, et al. Transanal minimal invasive surgery for rectal lesions: should the defect be closed? Color Dis. 2015;17:397–402.
23. Atallah S, Drake J, Martin-Perez B, Kang C, Larach S. Robotic transanal total mesorectal excision with intersphincteric dissection for extreme distal rectal cancer: a video demonstration. Tech Coloproctol. 2015;19:435.
24. Hompes R, Rauh SM, Ris F, Tuynman JB, Mortensen NJ. Robotic transanal minimally invasive surgery for local excision of rectal neoplasms. Br J Surg. 2014;101:578–81.
25. Xu ZS, Cheng H, Xiao Y, Cao JQ, Cheng F, et al. Comparison of transanal endoscopic microsurgery with or without neoadjuvant therapy and standard total mesorectal excision in the treatment of clinical T2 low rectal cancer: a meta-analysis. Oncotarget. 2017;8:115681–90.
26. Borstlap WA, Tanis PJ, Koedam TW, Marijnen CA, Cunningham C, et al. A multi-centred randomised trial of radical surgery versus adjuvant chemoradiotherapy after local excision for early rectal cancer. BMC Cancer. 2016;16:513.
27. Plummer JM, Leake PA, Albert MR. Recent advances in the management of rectal cancer: no surgery, minimal surgery or minimally invasive surgery. World J Gastrointest Surg. 2017;9:139–48.
28. Eid Y, Alves A, Lubrano J, Menahem B. Does previous transanal excision for early rectal cancer impair surgical outcomes and pathologic findings of completion total mesorectal excision? Results of a systematic review of the literature. J Visc Surg. 2018;155:445–52.
29. Letarte F, Raval M, Karimuddin A, Phang PT, Brown CJ. Salvage TME following TEM: a possible indication for TaTME. Tech Coloproctol. 2018;22:355–61.
30. Marks JH, Valsdottir EB, DeNittis A, Yarandi SS, Newman DA, et al. Transanal endoscopic microsurgery for the treatment of rectal cancer: comparison of wound complication rates with and without neoadjuvant radiation therapy. Surg Endosc. 2009;23:1081–7.
31. Perez RO, Habr-Gama A, Sao Juliao GP, Proscurshim I, Scanavini Neto A, et al. Transanal endoscopic microsurgery for residual rectal cancer after neoadjuvant chemoradiation therapy is associated with significant immediate pain and hospital readmission rates. Dis Colon Rectum. 2011;54:545–51.
32. Caycedo-Marulanda A, Jiang HY, Kohtakangas EL. Transanal minimally invasive surgery for benign large rectal polyps and early malignant rectal cancers: experience and outcomes from the first Canadian Centre to adopt the technique. Can J Surg. 2017;60:416–23.
33. Karakayali FY, Tezcaner T, Moray G. Anorectal function and outcomes after transanal minimally invasive surgery for rectal tumors. J Minim Access Surg. 2015;11:257–62.
34. Verseveld M, Barendse RM, Gosselink MP, Verhoef C, de Graaf EJ, et al. Transanal minimally invasive surgery: impact on quality of life and functional outcome. Surg Endosc. 2016;30:1184–7.

35. Burke JP, Atallah S, Albert MR. Transanal endoscopic resection with peritoneal entry: a word of reason. Tech Coloproctol. 2015;19:663–4.
36. Molina G, Bordeianou L, Shellito P, Sylla P. Transanal endoscopic resection with peritoneal entry: a word of caution. Surg Endosc. 2016;30:1816–25.
37. Salm R, Lampe H, Bustos A, Matern U. Experience with TEM in Germany. Endosc Surg Allied Technol. 1994;2:251–4.
38. Keller DS, Tahilramani RN, Flores-Gonzalez JR, Mahmood A, Haas EM. Transanal minimally invasive surgery: review of indications and outcomes from 75 consecutive patients. J Am Coll Surg. 2016;222:814–22.
39. Martin-Perez B, Andrade-Ribeiro GD, Hunter L, Atallah S. A systematic review of transanal minimally invasive surgery (TAMIS) from 2010 to 2013. Tech Coloproctol. 2014;18:775–88.
40. Schiphorst AH, Langenhoff BS, Maring J, Pronk A, Zimmerman DD. Transanal minimally invasive surgery: initial experience and short-term functional results. Dis Colon Rectum. 2014;57:927–32.
41. Arezzo A, Passera R, Saito Y, Sakamoto T, Kobayashi N, et al. Systematic review and meta-analysis of endoscopic submucosal dissection versus transanal endoscopic microsurgery for large noninvasive rectal lesions. Surg Endosc. 2014;28:427–38.
42. Atallah S, Albert M, Debeche-Adams T, Larach S. Transanal minimally invasive surgery (TAMIS): applications beyond local excision. Tech Coloproctol. 2013;17:239–43.
43. Atallah S, Martin-Perez B, Parra-Davila E, deBeche-Adams T, Nassif G, et al. Robotic transanal surgery for local excision of rectal neoplasia, transanal total mesorectal excision, and repair of complex fistulae: clinical experience with the first 18 cases at a single institution. Tech Coloproctol. 2015;19:401–10.
44. Ma B, Gao P, Song Y, Zhang C, Zhang C, et al. Transanal total mesorectal excision (taTME) for rectal cancer: a systematic review and meta-analysis of oncological and perioperative outcomes compared with laparoscopic total mesorectal excision. BMC Cancer. 2016;16:380.
45. Perdawood SK, Al Khefagie GA. Transanal vs laparoscopic total mesorectal excision for rectal cancer: initial experience from Denmark. Color Dis. 2016;18:51–8.
46. Fernandez-Hevia M, Delgado S, Castells A, Tasende M, Momblan D, et al. Transanal total mesorectal excision in rectal cancer: short-term outcomes in comparison with laparoscopic surgery. Ann Surg. 2015;61:221–7.
47. Velthuis S, Nieuwenhuis DH, Ruijter TE, Cuesta MA, Bonjer HJ, et al. Transanal versus traditional laparoscopic total mesorectal excision for rectal carcinoma. Surg Endosc. 2014;28:3494–9.
48. Denost Q, Adam JP, Rullier A, Buscail E, Laurent C, et al. Perineal transanal approach: a new standard for laparoscopic sphincter-saving resection in low rectal cancer, a randomized trial. Ann Surg. 2014;260:993–9.
49. Deijen CL, Velthuis S, Tsai A, Mavroveli S, de Lange-de Klerk ES, et al. COLOR III: a multicentre randomised clinical trial comparing transanal TME versus laparoscopic TME for mid and low rectal cancer. Surg Endosc. 2016;30:3210–5.

Chapter 10
Transanal Total Mesorectal Excision

Emeka Ray-Offor and Victor Strassmann

Introduction

The concept of total mesorectal excision (TME) was a landmark innovation for the surgery of rectal cancer in the past four decades [1]. The minimally invasive option of laparoscopic rectal surgery is widely reported to have no differences in oncological outcomes when compared with open procedures [2, 3]. Achieving an optimal TME with in-line rigid instruments from angles that require complicated maneuvers to reach the extremes of the pelvis is challenging during the resection of low rectal tumors. Transanal total mesorectal excision (taTME) is a "bottom-up" approach that has been developed from previous experience from a combination of techniques; transanal endoscopic microsurgery, transanal transabdominal approach to TME, single incision laparoscopic surgery and transanal minimally invasive surgery. This concept, developed in experimental models, was first described in a patient by Sylla et al. in 2010 [4].

The surgical technique of taTME facilitates direct intraluminal vision of rectal wall transection and surgical planes (mesorectum, autonomic nerves, and surrounding structures) providing a good quality of TME specimen and sphincter complex preservation. A direct visualization permits safe dissection around the vital

---

E. Ray-Offor (✉)
College of Health Sciences, University of Port Harcourt, Choba,
Rivers State, Nigeria

Colorectal/Minimal Access Surgery Unit, Department of Surgery, University of Port Harcourt Teaching Hospital, Port Harcourt, Rivers State, Nigeria
e-mail: emeka.ray-offor@uniport.edu.ng

V. Strassmann
Department of Colorectal Surgery, Ellen Leifer Shulman and Steven Shulman Digestive Disease Institute, Cleveland Clinic Florida, Weston, FL, USA

© The Author(s), under exclusive license to Springer Nature Switzerland AG 2024
E. Ray-Offor, R. J. Rosenthal (eds.), *Colorectal & Hernia Laparoscopic Surgery*, https://doi.org/10.1007/978-3-031-63490-1_10

structures that encircle the narrow pelvis, including the vagina, prostate, and pelvic neurovascular structures [5]. There is the avoidance of multiple firing of stapler in standard anterior resection which has a high risk of anastomotic leak. Also, natural orifice specimen extraction is facilitated by taTME with the potential for decreased surgical site infection and abdominal wall hernias. Despite conflicting reports of its long-term oncological outcomes, surgical centers across the world have adopted it into the armamentarium of surgical options for rectal cancer treatment [6–12].

Indications

The indications to perform taTME are primarily MRI-defined distal rectal cancers [13]. A consensus on indications of taTME by experts recommended this bottom-up TME approach for patients with the following characteristics: male, narrow and deep pelvis, obese, tumor less than 4 cm from the anal verge, prostate enlargement, and distorted planes caused by irradiation [14].

Ultra-Low Rectal Tumors

Patients who have low rectal tumors with a distal margin of 1–2 cm near the dentate line and not involving the sphincter complex are suited for sphincter preservation surgery by taTME. The lower margin of the tumor is identified under direct vision in the perianal stage of the procedure. Intersphincteric resection with coloanal anastomoses is facilitated by taTME [15].

Obesity

Surgery is often challenging in the presence of dense intrabdominal fat in patients with a high body mass index. This may obscure the visualization of anatomical landmarks with the attendant risk of unfavorable grade of TME surgery. The two-team approach of taTME can reduce the TME time compared to conventional laparoscopic low anterior resection.

Narrow and Deep Pelvis

Conventional laparoscopic low anterior resection is challenging in patients with narrow and deep pelvis more so with bulky distal rectal tumours. The difficult introduction of instruments with a limited range of movement in the pelvis is an obstacle that favors the choice of taTME.

Technical Difficulty

Surgeons beyond the learning curve of taTME offer this surgical technique in conditions where scarring and/or adhesions are likely to be encountered like patients with a history of pelvic surgery (e.g., prostatectomy; previous pelvic radiation (other than neoadjuvant therapy); and completion TME after a previous full-thickness local excision.

Others

Additionally, taTME has potential benefits in non-malignant conditions including reversal of Hartmann procedure, restorative proctocolectomy or completion proctectomy and ileal-pouch anal anastomosis (IPAA), and abdominoperineal resection (APR) [16].

Contraindications

Patients with clinical stage 4 tumors, tumors invading the sphincter complex, and tumors with a predicted positive circumferential margin (CRM+) with no evidence of significant post-treatment response on restaging MRI are not ideal candidates for taTME. In these settings, an APR (standard or extralevator) and anterior exenteration involving en bloc resection of vagina/ prostatectomy ± posterior exenteration involving sacral bone to achieve R0 resection are considered surgical options.

Preoperative Preparation

A complete evaluation of rectal cancer patients with preoperative staging based on accepted guidelines is adopted in all cases as earlier described for laparoscopic anterior resection in Chap. 5. Ideally, the management plan is discussed in a multidisciplinary meeting. A preoperative visit to the stoma therapist is at the surgeon's discretion. Bowel preparation and thromboprophylaxis are necessary. An informed consent is obtained from the patient providing information on other options of treatment and the risk of surgery. Preparation for surgery is conducted according to enhanced recovery after surgery guidelines.

The requisite instruments are 2 separate operating sets for the abdominal and perineal fields. This comprises two laparoscopy sets with two sets of optical devices (10 mm or 5 mm, 30 ° or 0 °, and 3D), two CO_2 insufflation systems, two energy device sets, two aspirators, two boxes of the basic instruments required for placement of trocars, removal of the specimen and anastomosis [17]. A short linear endostapler with different sizes of cartridges depending on the type of anastomosis (end-to-side, colonic J pouch) are needed for transabdominal colon transection. Also needed are tables for laparoscopic instruments and two Mayo tables for basic instruments. The trays for the perineal field comprise a soft TAMIS platform (e.g., Gelpoint Applied Medical, SILS Medtronic) (Fig. 10.1) with an operating anoscope, insufflating device, and an anal retractor. Rigid platforms of TEMS and TEO may be used. The energy device for transanal surgery is a monopolar L-hook electrode and bipolar coagulating instrument. For mechanical anastomosis, a transanal circular endostapler (size 28, 31, or 33 mm) and a circular hemorrhoidal stapler are needed.

Anesthesia

General anesthesia with deep neuromuscular blockade is performed and an endotracheal intubation is achieved.

Positioning

The two-team sequential approach is hereby described. At the start of surgery, the patient is in a modified lithotomy position. The arms are tucked to the patient's side and legs in stirrups. A secure strap is applied to the chest region. The abdominal surgeon and camera operator are positioned on the patient's right side and the other assistant surgeon on the opposite side of the table.

Fig. 10.1 TAMIS platform and insufflation tubing

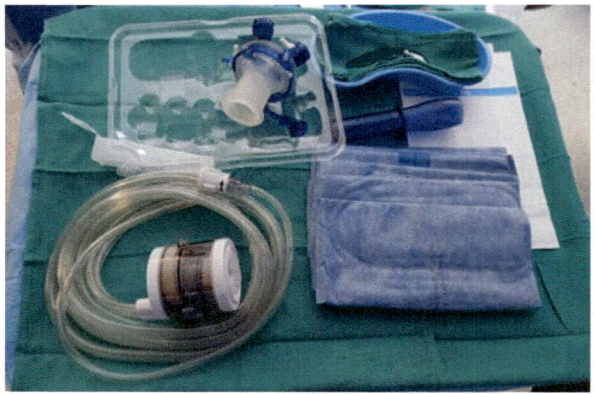

Technique

In settings where fluorescence image-guided technology is available a cystoscopy is performed by a Urologist with insertion of bilateral ureteric catheters and an injection of 5 cc of fluorescence dye into each ureter. A Foley catheter is inserted with a connecting bridge for the stents attached. A mushroom-tipped Malecot catheter is placed in the rectum through which approximately 1 L of normal saline is irrigated until the effluent is clear. Betadine is then introduced in the catheter and the catheter is left taped inside a plastic bag. The abdomen and perineum are cleaned and draped in the usual sterile manner.

Port Placement

An optical 10 mm port is inserted in a midline supraumbilical site using an open-access Hasson method. Capnoperitoneum of 12–15 mmHg is created and maintained. Three working ports are created by the insertion of trocars in the right flank, right iliac, and left iliac fossae under direct vision. In the presence of a previous laparotomy scar, primary access is achieved through a subcostal port in the left midclavicular line followed by the supraumbilical port under direct vision and transfer of camera to the latter. A medial traction is applied to the sigmoid colon and the lateral left colonic attachment to the lateral abdominal wall is dissected in a lateral-to-medial approach in the plane anterior to the Gerota fascia and retroperitoneal structures. Care is taken to identify the left ureter with the aid of fluorescence angiography and pushing it downwards and out of the dissection plane. Next, the omentum is tented, and a cut is made into the lesser sac away from the epiploic vessel, and subsequent dissection continues towards the splenic flexure. With a combined dissection along the line of Toldt towards the spleen, the splenic flexure is mobilized. Lateral traction on the sigmoid mesentery is then applied to identify the inferior mesenteric vessels and the peritoneum is opened to expose the plane anterior to retroperitoneal tissues. The inferior mesenteric artery is ligated about a centimeter away from its origin from the aorta with a vessel-sealing device. Caudally, at the level of the inferior border of the pancreas, the inferior mesenteric vein is visualized and ligated in the same fashion. A circumferential pelvic dissection is done starting posteriorly and progressing distally, laterally then anteriorly until it becomes difficult due to poor exposure. The abdominal phase is then paused after clamping off the sigmoid colon.

Transanal Phase

Self-retaining anal retractor (Lonestar, Cooper Surgical, Trumbull, CT, USA) is used to open the anus and identify the dentate line. Anal dilators are used for an atraumatic introduction of the transanal platform. Tumour is reassessed for distance from the anal verge (Fig. 10.2a and b).

The wide trocar of the TAMIS platform is inserted in an inverted triangle fashion and the cap with optical and working trocars at 11, 7, and 5 o'clock positions is applied (Fig. 10.3). Pneumorectum is created to a pressure of 12–15 mmHg preceded by the reduction of pneumoperitoneum pressure to 10 mmHg. This aids transanal dissection. An airtight purse string is created distal to the tumor to close off the rectal lumen using 0 polypropylene suture on a 26-mm rounded needle. Care is taken to take similar-sized bites of tissue at the same distance around the circumference of the lumen. The rectal mucosa, just distal to the mucosal folds formed by the purse string, is circumferentially tattooed with a hook electrode. A full-thickness perpendicular transection of the rectal wall is done with the monopolar hook. A sharp 'bottom-up' dissection is started following the avascular plane between the visceral and parietal fasciae of the pelvis and avoiding a cone shape or an excessive lateral dissection outside the safe plane. Dissection is continued proximally posteriorly between the posterior mesorectum and presacral fascia. In the lateral plane, care is taken not to veer into the pelvic sidewall resulting in problematic bleeding. Anteriorly, the dissection is performed in the plane between the rectal wall and rectovaginal or recto-prostatic fascia. This circumferential dissection with coordinated joint dissection is continued to the rendezvous point when both fields communicate and the rectosigmoid is completely dissected free. The specimen is extracted transabdominal in case of bulky tumors or narrow pelvis, or by transanal route.

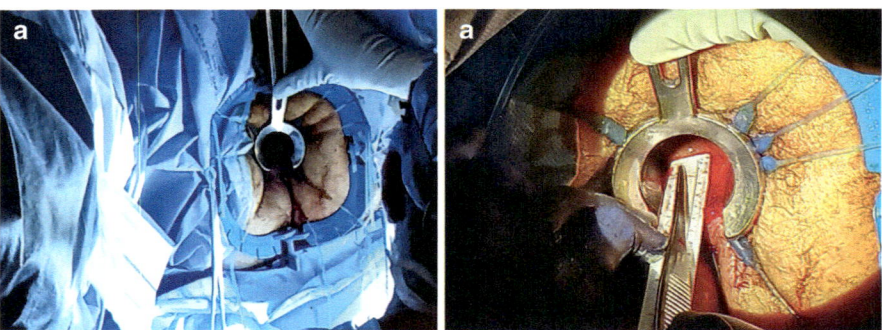

Fig. 10.2 (**a**) Anal inspection. (**b**) On-table assessment of tumour from anal verge

Fig. 10.3 Transanal platform in place

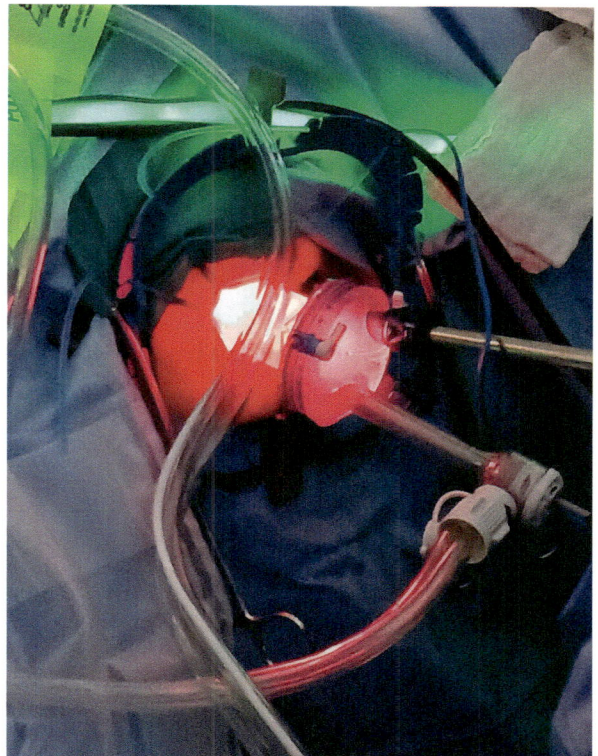

Anastomosis

Before bowel transection, the extracted specimen perfusion is assessed using indocyanine green dye (ICG). A handsewn or stapled anastomosis can be performed based on the distance of the transected rectal margin from the dentate line depending on the tumor distance from the anal verge and the resulting rectal stump length. For a stapled anastomosis, an adequate cut edge of the distal rectum must be mobilized for the purse string to be applied. The anvil is inserted and secured inside the proximal colon and returned to the pelvis by the appropriate surgical team depending on whether the extraction was done by transabdominal or transabdominal route. The distal purse string suture is applied using a 33-mm circular haemorrhoidal stapler and is closed and tied to the rod of the circular stapler. The anvil and rod of the circular stapler are connected, and the stapler is fired. After firing, the transanal platform is reinserted to verify the anastomosis for bleeding and completeness. Additional sutures can be placed to reinforce the anastomosis as needed. For a handsewn technique, commonly four reference sutures are made to the distal rectal stump and then passed through the proximal colon wall at the distal margin (end-to-end) or margin of a created colotomy in the antimesenteric border (end-to-side). The colon is well aligned without tension or twisting, and anastomosis is completed with simple stitches of 3–0 polyglycolic acid.

The abdominal cavity is inspected for proper hemostasis and a diverting ileostomy is made in high-risk patients: previously irradiated, colo-anal anastomosis, obese, or with other risk factors. A close-suction drainage is placed in the pelvis. Abdominal incisions are closed in a regular fashion.

Postoperative Care

Resected specimens are sent for histopathology. ERAS protocol is applied with early mobilization and feeding. Removal of the catheter is delayed to day 3 post-op in males with enlarged prostate and known risk factors of urinary retention. Discharge criteria include tolerating oral feeds, good stoma function, and nil untoward complications.

Special Notes

Like every novel surgical technique, further subjection to scientific scrutiny is needed [18–20]. The international taTME registry reports an anastomotic failure rate of 15.7% with independent risk factors including male sex, obesity, smoking, diabetes mellitus, tumors>25 mm, excessive intraoperative blood loss, manual anastomosis, and prolonged perineal operative time [21]. Additionally reported is a pelvic abscess rate of 4.7%, an anastomotic fistula rate of 0.8%, a chronic sinus rate of 0.9%, and an anastomotic stricture rate of 3.6%. There are significant reports of urethral injuries ranging from <1% to 11% in the literature [22]. Despite these, taTME is associated with clear technical benefits over conventional laparoscopic low anterior resection; demonstrated in male, obese low rectal cancer male patients with a narrow pelvis [23]. Evidence from randomized controlled study demonstrates a lower conversion rate in taTME than conventional laparoscopic total mesorectal excision in centers with experienced surgeons [24]. Experienced surgeons can safely perform taTME in selected patients with rectal cancer with no difference in intraoperative complication, postoperative morbidity, and mortality [25]. In all, taTME is a useful tool in the surgeon's armamentarium for the management of distal rectal cancer.

References

1. Heald RJ, Husband EM, Ryall RD. The mesorectum in rectal cancer surgery—the clue to pelvic recurrence? Br J Surg. 1982;69:613–6.
2. van der Pas MH, Haglind E, Cuesta MA, Fürst A, Lacy AM, Hop WC, et al. Laparoscopic versus open surgery for rectal cancer (COLOR II): short-term outcomes of a randomised, phase 3 trial. Lancet Oncol. 2013;14:210–8.
3. Bonjer HJ, Deijen CL, Abis GA, Cuesta MA, van der Pas MH, de Lange-de Klerk ES, et al. A randomized trial of laparoscopic versus open surgery for rectal cancer. N Engl J Med. 2015;372:1324–32.
4. Sylla P, Rattner DW, Delgado S, Lacy AM. NOTES transanal rectal cancer resection using transanal endoscopic microsurgery and laparoscopic assistance. Surg Endosc. 2010;24:1205–10.
5. de Lacy AM, Rattner DW, Adelsdorfer C, Tasende MM, Fernandez M, Delgado S, et al. Transanal natural orifice transluminal endoscopic surgery (NOTES) rectal resection: "down-to-up" total mesorectal excision (TME)–short-term outcomes in the first 20 cases. Surg Endosc. 2013;27(9):3165–72.
6. Jiang HP, Li YS, Wang B, Wang C, Liu F, Shen ZL, et al. Pathological outcomes of transanal versus laparoscopic total mesorectal excision for rectal cancer: a systematic review with meta-analysis. Surg Endosc. 2018;32:2632–42.
7. Caycedo-Marulanda A, Lee L, Chadi SA, Verschoor CP, Crosina J, Ashamalla S, et al. Association of transanal total mesorectal excision with local recurrence of rectal cancer. JAMA Netw Open. 2021;4(2):e2036330.
8. Roodbeen SX, Spinelli A, Bemelman WA, Di Candido F, Cardepont M, Denost Q, et al. Local recurrence after transanal total mesorectal excision for rectal cancer: a multicenter cohort study. Ann Surg. 2021;274(2):359–66.
9. Trépanier JS, Fernandez-Hevia M, Lacy AM. Transanal total mesorectal excision: surgical technique description and outcomes. Minim Invasive Ther Allied Technol. 2016;25:234–40.
10. Moon JY, Lee MR, Ha GW. Long-term oncologic outcomes of transanal TME compared with transabdominal TME for rectal cancer: a systematic review and metanalysis. Surg Endosc. 2022;36(5):3122–35.
11. Denost Q, Loughlin P, Chevalier R, Celerier B, Didailler R, Rullier E. Transanal versus abdominal low rectal dissection for rectal cancer: long-term results of the Bordeaux' randomized trial. Surg Endosc. 2018;32:1486–94.
12. Hol JC, van Oostendorp SE, Tuynman JB, Sietses C. Long-term oncological results after transanal total mesorectal excision for rectal carcinoma. Tech Coloproctol. 2019;23:903–11.
13. Shwaartz C, Sylla P. Transanal total mesorectal excision. Chapter. In: Wexner SD, Fleshman JW, editors. Colon and rectal surgery. 2nd ed. Philadelphia, PA: Wolters Kluwer; 2019. p. 187–210.
14. Motson RW, Whiteford MH, Hompes R, Albert M, Miles WF, Expert Group. Current status of trans-anal total mesorectal excision (TaTME) following the Second International Consensus Conference. Color Dis. 2016;18(1):13–8.
15. Varela C, Kim NK. Surgical treatment of low-lying rectal cancer: updates. Ann Coloproctol. 2021;37(6):395–424.
16. D'Andrea AP, McLemore EC, Bonaccorso A, Cuevas JM, Basam M, Tsay AT, et al. Transanal total mesorectal excision (taTME) for rectal cancer: beyond the learning curve. Surg Endosc. 2020;34(9):4101–9.
17. Arroyave MC, DeLacy FB, Lacy AM. Transanal total mesorectal excision (TaTME) for rectal cancer: step-by-step description of the surgical technique for a two-team approach. Eur J Surg Oncol. 2017 Feb;43(2):502–5.
18. An Y, Roodbeen SX, Talboom K, Tanis PJ, Bemelman WA, Hompes R. A systematic review and meta-analysis on complications of transanal total mesorectal excision. Color Dis. 2021;23:2527–38.

19. Munini M, Popeskou SG, Galetti K, Roesel R, Mongelli F, Christoforidis D. Transanal (TaTME) vs. laparoscopic total mesorectal excision for mid and low rectal cancer: a propensity score-matched analysis of early and long-term outcomes. Int J Color Dis. 2021;36:2271–9.
20. Hallam S, Ahmed F, Gouvas N, Pandey S, Nicol D. Oncological outcomes and stoma-free survival following TaTME, a prospective cohort study. Tech Coloproctol. 2021;25:439–47.
21. Penna M, Hompes R, Arnold S, Wynn G, Austin R, Warusavitarne J, et al. Incidence and risk factors for anastomotic failure in 1594 patients treated by transanal total mesorectal excision: results from the international TaTME registry. Ann Surg. 2019;269:700–11.
22. Sylla P, Knol JJ, D'Andrea AP, Perez RO, Atallah SB, Penna M, et al. Urethral injury and other urologic injuries during transanal total mesorectal excision: an international collaborative study. Ann Surg. 2021;274:e1.
23. Mizrahi I, Sands DR. Transanal total mesorectal excision for rectal cancer: a review. Ann Laparosc Endosc Surg. 2017;2:14.
24. Serra-Aracil X, Zarate A, Bargalló J, Gonzalez A, Serracant A, Roura J, Delgado S, Mora-López L, Ta-LaTME study Group. Transanal versus laparoscopic total mesorectal excision for mid and low rectal cancer (Ta-LaTME study): a multicentre, randomized, open-label trial. Br J Surg. 2023;110(2):150–8.
25. Liu H, Zeng Z, Zhang H, Wu M, Ma D, Wang Q, et al. Chinese Transanal Endoscopic Surgery Collaborative (CTESC) Group. Morbidity, mortality, and pathologic outcomes of transanal versus laparoscopic total mesorectal excision for rectal cancer short-term outcomes from a multicenter randomized controlled trial. Ann Surg. 2023;277(1):1–6.

Part III
Pelvic Floor

Chapter 11
Laparoscopic Ventral Rectopexy

Mukhtar Ahmad

Introduction

Ventral Rectopexy (VR) is a surgical procedure that involves securing the rectum and vagina to the sacral promontory using synthetic mesh or biologic implant. Abdominal rectopexy has been described since the 1950s as an open operation but the history of laparoscopic rectopexy can be traced back to the development of laparoscopic surgery in the late 1980s and early 1990s. In recent years, laparoscopic rectopexy has been further advanced with robot-assisted surgical systems. Robotic surgery allows for enhanced precision and dexterity, making it particularly useful for complex procedures like rectopexy.

The first laparoscopic rectopexy procedure is attributed to Dr. James W. Fleshman and his team at Baylor University Medical Center in Dallas, Texas, in 1990. Andre D'Hoore first described the current iteration of laparoscopic ventral rectopexy [1]. Various modifications have been made to the technique over the years. Different methods of securing the rectum, such as sutures, mesh, or a combination of both, have been used. The choice of technique depends on the surgeon's preference and the patient's characteristics.

Overall, laparoscopic rectopexy has become an established surgical option for the treatment of internal and external rectal prolapse [2]. It has provided patients with a less invasive alternative to open surgery, resulting in reduced morbidity, faster recovery, and improved quality of life. However, as with any surgical procedure, the decision to perform laparoscopic rectopexy should be made on a case-by-case basis, considering the patient's circumstances and the surgeon's expertise. Multidisciplinary team discussion is recommended before a decision is made to offer surgery.

M. Ahmad (✉)
University Hospitals, Dorset, UK
mukhtar.ahmad@uhd.nhs.uk

Relevant Anatomy

- The levator ani is a conglomeration of several small muscles that together form the pelvic floor (see Fig. 6.1 of Chap. 6). Damage to these muscles during childbirth or weakening because of menopause and the aging process allows the pelvic floor to descend excessively. This is described as excessive perineal descent measured from the pubococcygeal line.
- The hypogastric nerves are at risk of damage during dissection as they splay over the sacral promontory towards the pelvic side wall.
- The ureter is at risk during the lateral peritoneal dissection and closure of the peritoneal defect.
- Avoid denuding the rectum laterally to reduce the likelihood of damage to the nerve supply.
- Avoid dissecting below the prostate and seminal vesicles to avoid damaging the *Nervi erigentes*.

Indications

External rectal prolapse
    Internal Rectal Prolapse (Rectoanal intussusception)
    Solitary Rectal Ulcer Syndrome

Contra-Indications

1. Pregnancy
2. Absence of pelvic anatomical derangement
3. Severe intra-abdominal adhesions
4. Active proctitis
5. Psychological instability
6. Anismus (paradoxical contraction of the puborectalis) resistant to conventional treatment

Pre-operative Preparation

- Colonoscopy or flexible sigmoidoscopy (FIT test would suffice in the absence of any concerning symptoms)
- Proctogram
    - MRI

- Fluoroscopy
- Endoanal USS
- Anorectal physiology
- Urodynamics (if significant urinary symptoms)
- Examination under anesthetic if doubt remains after the above investigations
- MDT discussion

On Admission

- A phosphate enema should be given on admission.
- Broad-spectrum antibiotics should be given at induction.

Anesthesia

General anesthesia is required for all laparoscopic procedures. Spinal anesthesia could be considered in addition to post-operative analgesia but this is not mandatory. The drawback of spinal anesthesia is the requirement to leave an indwelling bladder catheter until the spinal anesthetic has worn off. The author has found instillation of local anesthetic into the pelvis and pre-peritoneal infiltration of the port sites provides adequate pain control in addition to simple oral analgesics.

Positioning (Fig. 11.1)

The patient is placed in the Lloyd-Davies position with the legs in hydraulic supports. A bladder catheter is inserted and can be removed at the end of the procedure if a spinal anesthetic has not been used. A non-slip mat, shoulder supports, or both should be used to reduce the likelihood of the patient sliding when the head-down position is adopted. The arms should be tucked in by the side to allow a comfortable position for the surgeon and assistants.

Access

Establish peritoneum using the open cutdown (Hasson) technique or Veress needle depending on your training and experience. Establish pneumoperitoneum maintaining the pressure between 9–12 mmHg. Insert the 5 mm and 10–12 mm ports in the positions shown in diagram 1. Consider using ports with retention balloons to

Fig. 11.1 Theatre set up

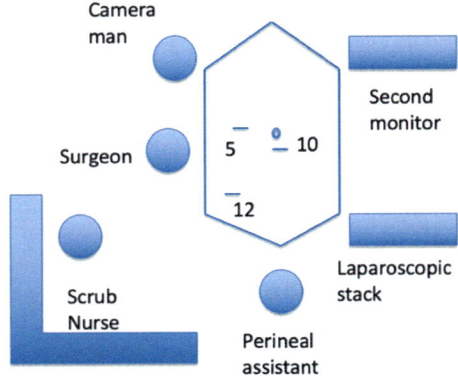

reduce the likelihood of displacement. An additional 5 mm port can be inserted in the left iliac fossa to aid retraction of the sigmoid colon.

Step-By-Step

Module 1

- Retraction
    - Retract the sigmoid colon towards the left using one of the following methods
        - Using a tacking device through the appendices epiploicae
        - Using a ligature e.g. Endoloop on the appendices epiploicae retrieved through a stab incision in the left LIF
        - Additional 5 mm port in the LIF
    - Insert a curved retractor such as a Kelly or Deaver into the vaginal fornix and ask the perineal assistant to lever the retractor backward lifting the vagina away from the rectum, aiding the dissection of the rectovaginal septum. Purpose-made vaginal retractors are also available
    - A rectal sizer can be used in the rectum to identify the lateral edges of the rectum and maneuver it during suturing

Module 2

- Peritoneal dissection
    - Holding up the peritoneum over the sacral promontory, make an incision using monopolar diathermy

- Continue along the right border of the rectum taking care not to damage the ureter on the right pelvic sidewall and the hypogastric nerves and stopping short of the pelvic floor
- Grasp the peritoneum in the deepest recess of the Pouch of Douglas and commence another incision continuing to the anorectal junction. This can be identified by the median raphe and digital examination. In a male, dissection should stop at the prostate, and lateral dissection should be avoided to reduce the likelihood of damaging the nervi erigentes
- Connect the two incisions and deepen the lateral incision to allow the biologic implant or mesh adequate space to line in

Module 3

Mesh Fixation

Secure the mesh to the ventral surface of the rectum, posterior wall of the vagina, and sacral promontory as described below. Biologic implants are currently preferred because of the heightened awareness of mesh erosion. Though historically, biologic implants have been associated with higher recurrence rates, series from specialist centers have shown that lower recurrence rates could be achieved [3].

- Rectum and vagina
  - Prepare the mesh/ implant.

    The mesh should ideally be 18-20 cm long and 4 cm wide. Synthetic or biologic implants could be used taking into account increased risk of complications with the former and higher recurrence rates with the latter.
    Draw a line across one end of the mesh 2 cm from the edge—your first sutures should be passed through this line to ensure there is a flange of mesh to suture to the anorectal junction when the mesh is secured to the sacral promontory
    Cut a 0.5 cm strip off the left border of the mesh starting at the sacral promontory end curving towards the middle of the mesh. This step prevents constriction
  - Use a slowly absorbable suture such as 2–0 PDS to attach the mesh to the rectum and vaginal vault/ posterior fornix or paracervical fascia. Place the first sutures on both lateral edges of the rectum just above the anorectal junction. Place more sutures on both edges of the rectum making sure to straighten the rectum and the mesh each time to prevent an iatrogenic kink
  - Sacral promontory

After the first four sutures, secure the tail of the mesh to the sacral promontory using a non-absorbable suture such as Ethibond or tacking devices such as Protack.

Module 4

Reperitonealisation

- Close the peritoneal defect using a continuous absorbable suture starting at the vaginal vault or posterior fornix (if the uterus is still in place)
- A barbed self-retaining suture could save time if this is available
- It might be necessary to perform a culdectomy (excising excess peritoneum in the Pouch of Douglas). Take care not to damage the rectum by using a rectal sizer to identify its edges.

Post-operative Care

- Low molecular weight heparin until discharge from hospital
- Early mobilization and discharge within 24 hours if well
- Day case procedure is feasible with adequate safety-netting.

Complications

- Haemorrhage
- Vaginal or rectal perforation
- Urinary retention (<10%)
- Worsening or de novo stress urinary incontinence
- Faecal impaction (rare)
- Male sexual dysfunction (rare)
- Dyspareunia (uncommon) usually resolves with time
- Osteomyelitis of the sacrum and spondylodiscitis (rare)
- Implant-related: infection, erosion, encasement

Special Notes

Potential Pitfalls

- Not dissecting down to the anorectal junction
- Too much tension when securing mesh to the promontory
- Not leaving an adequate flap to cover the bare distal rectum after sacral mobilization
- Not straightening rectum during mesh fixation

Recurrence

Though long-term data is limited, recurrence is thought to be higher with biologic implants.

Redo Surgery

Reoperating in the pelvis after rectopexy can be challenging because of the fibrosis that results from the implantation of synthetic or non-synthetic foreign material. The indications for redo surgery could include:

- Recurrence of prolapse
- Mesh erosion
- Mesh-related infection

Patients requiring revisional surgery should be referred to tertiary centers with expertise in this area.

References

1. D'Hoore A, Penninckx F. Laparoscopic ventral recto(colpo)pexy for rectal prolapse: surgical technique and outcome for 109 patients. Surg Endosc. 2006;20(12):1919–23.
2. Mercer-Jones MA, D'Hoore A, Dixon AR, Lehur P, Lindsey I, Mellgren A, Stevenson AR. Consensus on ventral rectopexy: report of a panel of experts. Color Dis. 2014;16(2):82–8.
3. Ahmad M, Sileri P, Franceschilli L, Mercer-Jones M. The role of biologics in pelvic floor surgery. Color Dis. 2012;14(Suppl 3):19–23.

Part IV
Hernia

Chapter 12
Laparoscopic Ventral Hernia Repair

Emeka Ray-Offor and Raul J. Rosenthal

Introduction

Primary and incisional ventral hernias are common indications for surgery worldwide with more than 350,000 ventral hernias repaired in the United States annually [1]. These are two different conditions with the latter being more challenging to treat. While primary ventral hernias are congenital and arising from adverse forces acting on the anterior abdominal wall, on the other hand, incisional hernia (IH) is any abdominal wall gap with or without a bulge around a postoperative scar perceptible or palpable by clinical examination or imaging [2]. IHs are one of the most common long-term complications that occur in 10–30% of laparotomy incisions and subsequent conventional open repair often leads to recurrence [3]. The recognized risk factors leading to hernia recurrence are preoperative (patient and hernia-related), intraoperative, and post-operative factors [4]. In all, the use of a mesh in primary ventral and incisional hernia repair lowers the recurrence rate and is the

---

E. Ray-Offor (✉)
College of Health Sciences, University of Port Harcourt, Choba, Rivers State, Nigeria

Colorectal/Minimal Access Surgery Unit, Department of Surgery, University of Port Harcourt Teaching Hospital, Port Harcourt, Rivers State, Nigeria
e-mail: emeka.ray-offor@uniport.edu.ng

R. J. Rosenthal
Ellen Leifer Shulman and Steven Shulman Digestive Disease Institute, Cleveland Clinic Florida, Weston, FL, USA

Division of General Surgery, Cleveland Clinic Florida, Weston, FL, USA

Cleveland Clinic Lerner College of Medicine at Case Western Reserve University, Cleveland, OH, USA

Charles E. Schmidt College of Medicine, Florida Atlantic University, Boca Raton, FL, USA

Herbert Wertheim College of Medicine, Florida International University, Miami, FL, USA

© The Author(s), under exclusive license to Springer Nature Switzerland AG 2024
E. Ray-Offor, R. J. Rosenthal (eds.), *Colorectal & Hernia Laparoscopic Surgery*, https://doi.org/10.1007/978-3-031-63490-1_12

accepted standard of care for larger defects [5]. Notably, the restoration of the abdominal wall anatomy by suturing the hernia aperture before mesh placement is not associated with an increased risk of hernia-site complication or chronic pain [6].

Traditionally, ventral hernia repair is performed by open technique but there is an increasing application of the laparoscopic technique which includes the extended totally extraperitoneal (eTEP) repair and intraperitoneal onlay mesh placement (IPOM) with or without prior suture approximation of defect [7]. Laparoscopic ventral hernia repair LVHR using the IPOM technique provides the additional benefit of a complete exploration of the abdominal cavity with a magnified view, the possibility to add another procedure if needed, and an easier adhesiolysis which is associated with a lower chronic postoperative abdominal pain [8]. Compared to open repair, LVHR has a comparable outcome but with a lower rate of surgical site infection SSI, post-operative pain, shorter hospital stays, albeit more recurrence [9–11]. Robot-assisted laparoscopic ventral hernia repair with intraperitoneal mesh has comparable outcomes with conventional LVHR but an increased operative time; the proportional cost of the robotic approach is not offset by a measurable clinical benefit [12, 13]. Hence a tailored approach for the repair of primary and incisional ventral hernia should be based on the surgeon's experience, clinical setting, patient's age and size, hernia defect size, and anatomical characteristics [14].

Different mesh fixation techniques are in use such as permanent tacks, absorbable tacks, and fibrin glue and suture fixation alone or in combination with tacks. Currently, none of the techniques in small- and medium-sized ventral hernias can be considered superior to another based on low or very low certainty of evidence for pain and recurrence [15, 16].

Relevant Anatomy

For the classification of ventral hernias, the abdomen is divided into medial or midline and lateral zones [2]. The borders of the medial zone are the xiphoid process cranially, pubic bone caudally, and the lateral margins of the rectus sheath on either side laterally. Primary ventral hernias located here are epigastric, umbilical, and paraumbilical. The classification of midline incisional is as follows: subxiphoidal M1- from the xiphoid process to 3 cm caudally; epigastric M2 from 3 cm below the xiphoid to 3 cm above the umbilicus; umbilical M3- from 3 cm above to 3 cm below the umbilicus; infraumbilical M4- from 3 cm below the umbilicus to 3 cm above the pubis; suprapubic M5- from pubic bone to 3 cm cranially [2].

For the lateral zone, the borders are the costal margin cranially, the inguinal region caudally, and laterally the lumbar region together with the lateral margin of the rectus sheath on either side of the lateral borders. The primary ventral hernias located laterally are the Spigelian and lumbar hernia. The classification of lateral zone incisional hernias is as follows: subcostal L1-between the costal margin and a horizontal line 3 cm above the umbilicus; Flank L2-lateral to the rectal sheath in the area 3 cm above and below the umbilicus; Iliac L3-between a horizontal line 3 cm below the umbilicus and the inguinal region; Lumbar L4-latero-dorsal of the anterior axillary line.

Indications and Contraindications

Generally, all ventral hernias can be repaired by a laparoscopic approach where the competence and equipment are available with due consideration given to the patient and hernia-related factors. LVHR is preferred in an elective setting for the following: (a) symptomatic ventral/incisional hernia larger than 3 cm; (b) recurrent hernia; (c) Immunocompromised [8, 17].

Absolute contraindications include ventral hernias having a defect of >20 cm associated with loss of domain and conditions with or prone to sepsis. In strangulated hernia, gangrenous bowel, peritonitis, intraabdominal sepsis, anterior abdominal skin infection, and enterocutaneous fistula, LVHR is not recommended [8]. Systemic conditions with risk of uncontrollable bleeding like cirrhosis with caput medusa are also contraindications for LVHR.

Preoperative Preparation

A full clinical examination including a history of previous abdominal surgeries and imaging is required to delineate the abdominal wall defect (length and width) and identify risk factors of hernia in addition to comorbidities for tailored surgical management. The length of the hernia defect is defined as the greatest vertical distance in cm between the most cranial and the most caudal margin of the hernia defect. In case of multiple hernia defects from one incision, the length is between the cranial margin of the most cranial defect and the caudal margin of the most caudal defect [2]. In elective surgery, preoperative behavioral modifications, with resultant weight loss, may reduce the effect of obesity [18]. Informed consent is obtained from the patient and for the patient's expectation management a careful explanation is made of the risks of surgery which may include enterotomy, seroma, conversion, recurrence, QoL related outcomes [19]. Bowel preparation is optional but antibiotic prophylaxis in the immediate preoperative period is mandatory. Deep vein thrombosis prophylaxis is required based on hospital/ local protocol.

A high-image quality laparoscopic set is essential in the operating room. The laparoscopic instruments needed include a 12 mm trocar for a 30-degree 10 mm laparoscope and insertion of mesh; two additional 5 mm working ports; a Veress needle is optional, but an optical trocar (Opti-View) is preferred. The 5 mm working instruments needed include atraumatic graspers, curved scissors, bowel clamp, suction/irrigation device, needle holder, suture passer, mesh fixation device (absorbable e.g. Absorba Tack or non-absorbable e.g. Pro Tack), and Prolene 0 suture. An appropriately sized mesh is required, and composite mesh is preferred e.g.,

DynaMesh®-IPOM, Parietex® (Covidien), and Vypro II (Ethicon). Also, an energy source is needed; diathermy and hook electrodes may be used if newer bipolar and ultrasonic energy devices are not available.

Technique

A laparoscopic IPOM repair of a small-sized ventral hernia is herein discussed. Transversus abdominis plane block significantly reduces both short-term postoperative opioid use and pain [20]. After successful induction of general endotracheal anesthesia with deep neuromuscular blockade, the patient is prepped in a standard supine position with both arms tucked at the side or on the arm board depending on the size and site of the hernia and draped in the usual sterile fashion. Time-out is called, the patient is correctly identified, and the procedure is clearly stated. Preoperative antibiotics are given and sequential compression devices and heparin injections are administered when indicated. The surgeon and assistant are positioned on the same side opposite the hernia side to enable an ideal half length of the laparoscopic instrument within the peritoneum for mechanical efficiency (the standard laparoscopic instrument is roughly 36 cm and about 45 cm for bariatric instruments).

A 2 cm incision is made in the left upper quadrant. Using the optical trocar, the abdominal cavity is accessed under direct visualization. An exploration of the abdominal cavity is made upon gaining access to exclude iatrogenic injuries during access creation, to identify defect(s) and any adhesion (Fig. 12.1).

Two 5-mm trocars are inserted in the left lower and left mid abdomen under direct visualization in a left sided approach. With the trocars away from the proximal edge of the hernia not to impede mesh overlap. At this point, the lysis of adhesions is done with the hernia sac emptied of its content (Fig. 12.2).

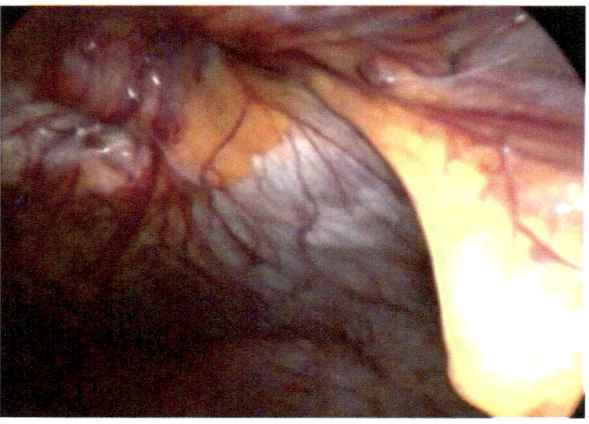

Fig. 12.1 Umbilical defect with adhesion

Fig. 12.2 Adhesiolysis

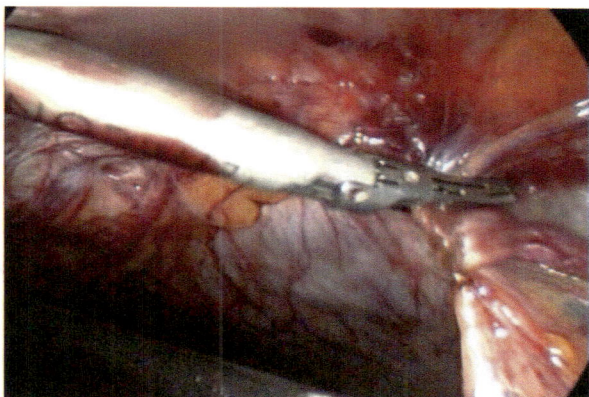

Fig. 12.3 Abdominal wall defect cleared of adhesions

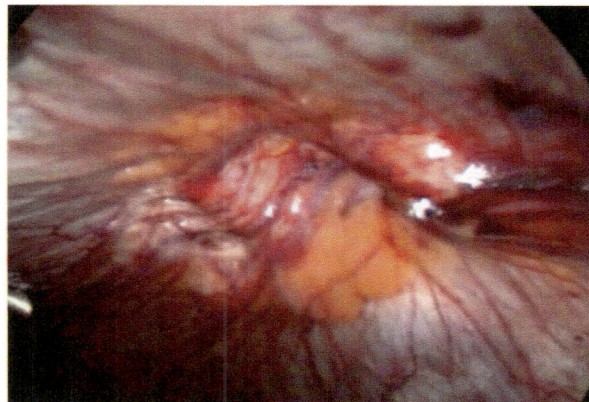

An external manipulation of the abdominal wall by the assistant may be needed to facilitate the emptying of the hernia sac. Care is taken not to use energy devices very close to the bowel. An enterotomy mandates an immediate repair and if there is gross spillage of intestinal content mesh repair can be delayed for 1–2 months. Dense adhesions of the bowel or incarcerated bowel may necessitate discontinuation and conversion to open surgery.

The abdominal wall defect now cleared of adhesion is measured by the introduction of a measuring tape or using a laparoscopic instrument with a predetermined distance between the open jaws (Fig. 12.3).

A reduction of capnoperitoneum to 8 mmHg at this instance is required. An external marking of the defect on the abdominal wall skin is helpful. The composite mesh is prepared with an overlap of 5 cm all around the defect. The composite mesh is tagged at four corners on the synthetic non-adhesive side with Prolene 0 suture and inked for orientation. The mesh is rolled on a laparoscopic instrument with a side for the parietal surface on the inside and introduced into the 12 mm trocar on withdrawal of the laparoscope. The mesh is unrolled and oriented within the abdomen. Using a suture passer oriented in different directions through a tiny stab wound at predetermined externally corresponding sites of mesh overlap, the sutures are exteriorized starting from the side furthest from the operating surgeon. All sutures are exteriorized before secure knots are made to facilitate proper orientation of the mesh. A mesh fixator (e.g. Protack, Absorba Tack) is inserted through one of the 5 mm ports and used to apply an external crown of tacks not more than 2 cm apart to avoid incarceration of the bowel in between the mesh and parietal surface (Figs. 12.4 and 12.5).

External pressure on the anterior abdominal wall is applied in the area being tacked to ensure it is well fastened to the fascia. An inner crown of tacks is then applied at the margin of the defect. A final inspection for hemostasis is made and the capnoperitoneum is released. Fascia closure of the 12 mm port site is made followed by subcuticular closure of all port sites. Local anesthetic is administered to transfascial suture sites with skin dressings and abdominal binder applied.

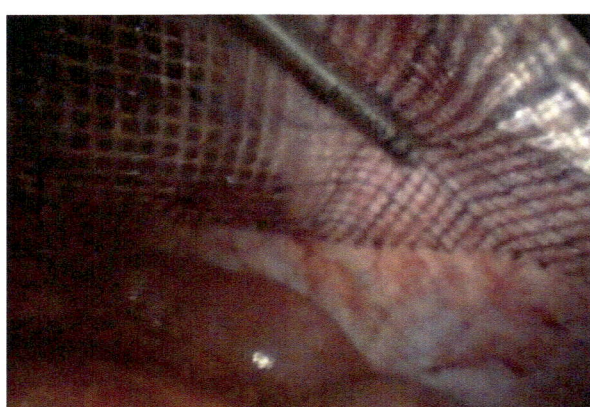

Fig. 12.4 Fixing mesh to the parietal fascia

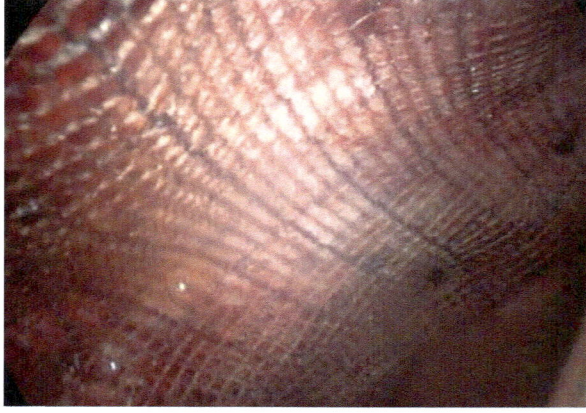

Fig. 12.5 Outer crown of tacks applied

Post-operative Care

Patients are encouraged to mobilize early. Abdominal binders are applied for 1 week as this practice is reported to promote wound healing, reduce pain, and prevent recurrent herniation after incisional hernia repair with the IPOM technique [21]. Early oral fluid intake is commenced 6–8 hours after surgery and graduated to solid food as tolerated. Analgesics are also administered. Usually, the patient is discharged home for outpatient visits 1–2 days after surgery in good clinical state. Notable complications are seroma, chronic pain (≥3 months after surgery) and recurrence. Closure of the fascial defect during LVHR can reduce the rate of seroma formation and adverse hernia-site events [22, 23].

Proper mesh overlap is a key determinant in hernia recurrence following laparoscopic ventral and incisional hernia repair. The risk of hernia recurrence is demonstrated to decrease with increasing area of mesh overlap in laparoscopic repair (<3 cm, incidence rate 0.086; 3–5 cm, incidence rate 0.046; >5 cm, incidence rate 0.014) [24].

References

1. Poulose BK, Shelton J, Phillips S, Moore D, Nealon W, Penson D, Beck W, Holzman MD. Epidemiology and cost of ventral hernia repair: making the case for hernia research. Hernia. 2012;16(2):179–83.
2. Muysoms FE, Miserez M, Berrevoet F, Campanelli G, Champault CG, Chelala E, et al. Classification of primary and incisional abdominal wall hernias. Hernia. 2009;13(4):407–14.
3. Mudge M, Hughes LE. Incisional hernia: a 10-year prospective study of incidence and attitudes. Br J Surg. 1985;72:70.
4. Parker SG, Mallett S, Quinn L, Wood CPJ, Boulton RW, Jamshaid S, et al. Identifying predictors of ventral hernia recurrence: systematic review and meta-analysis. BJS Open. 2021;5(2):zraa071.
5. Mathes T, Walgenbach M, Siegel R. Suture versus mesh repair in primary and incisional ventral hernias: a systematic review and meta-analysis. World J Surg. 2016;40(4):826–35.
6. Silfvenius AUK, Lindmark ME, Tall JV, Österberg JK, Strigård KK, Thorell A, Gunnarsson US. Laparoscopic ventral hernia repair: early follow-up of a randomized controlled study of primary fascial closure before mesh placement. Br J Surg. 2024;111(1):znad434.
7. Jain M, Krishna A, Prakash O, Kumar S, Sagar R, Ramachandran R, Bansal VK. Comparison of extended totally extra peritoneal (eTEP) vs intra peritoneal onlay mesh (IPOM) repair for management of primary and incisional hernia in terms of early outcomes and cost effectiveness-a randomized controlled trial. Surg Endosc. 2022;36(10):7494–502.
8. Malik S, Wijerrathne S. Laparoscopic intraperitoneal onlay mesh (IPOM) and IPOM plus. In: Lomanto D, Chen WTL, Fuentes MB, editors. Mastering endo-laparoscopic and thoracoscopic surgery. Singapore: Springer; 2023. p. 417–25.
9. Itani KM, Hur K, Kim LT, Anthony T, Berger DH, Reda D, Neumayer L, Veterans Affairs Ventral Incisional Hernia Investigators. Comparison of laparoscopic and open repair with mesh for the treatment of ventral incisional hernia: a randomized trial. Arch Surg. 2010;145(4):322–8. discussion 328

10. Arita NA, Nguyen MT, Nguyen DH, Berger RL, Lew DF, Suliburk JT, Askenasy EP, Kao LS, Liang MK. Laparoscopic repair reduces the incidence of surgical site infections for all ventral hernias. Surg Endosc. 2015;29(7):1769–80.
11. Asencio F, Carbó J, Ferri R, Peiró S, Aguiló J, Torrijo I, Barber S, Canovas R, Andreu-Ballester JC. Laparoscopic versus open incisional hernia repair: long-term follow-up results of a randomized clinical trial. World J Surg. 2021;45(9):2734–41.
12. Dhanani NH, Olavarria OA, Holihan JL, Shah SK, Wilson TD, Loor MM, Ko TC, Kao LS, Liang MK. Robotic versus laparoscopic ventral hernia repair: one-year results from a prospective, multicenter, blinded randomized controlled trial. Ann Surg. 2021;273(6):1076–80.
13. Petro CC, Zolin S, Krpata D, Alkhatib H, Tu C, Rosen MJ, Prabhu AS. Patient-reported outcomes of robotic vs laparoscopic ventral hernia repair with intraperitoneal mesh: the PROVE-IT randomized clinical trial. JAMA Surg. 2021;156(1):22–9.
14. Hajibandeh S, Hajibandeh S, Sreh A, Khan A, Subar D, Jones L. Laparoscopic versus open umbilical or paraumbilical hernia repair: a systematic review and meta-analysis. Hernia. 2017;21(6):905–16.
15. Mathes T, Prediger B, Walgenbach M, Siegel R. Mesh fixation techniques in primary ventral or incisional hernia repair. Cochrane Database Syst Rev. 2021;5(5):CD011563.
16. Harsløf S, Krum-Møller P, Sommer T, Zinther N, Wara P, Friis-Andersen H. Effect of fixation devices on postoperative pain after laparoscopic ventral hernia repair: a randomized clinical trial of permanent tacks, absorbable tacks, and synthetic glue. Langenbeck's Arch Surg. 2018;403(4):529–37.
17. Lambrecht JR, Skauby M, Trondsen E, Vaktskjold A, Øyen OM. Laparoscopic repair of incisional hernia in solid organ-transplanted patients: the method of choice? Transpl Int. 2014;27(7):712–20.
18. Sugerman H, Windsor A, Bessos M. Wolfe L intra-abdominal pressure, sagittal abdominal diameter, and obesity comorbidity. J Intern Med. 1997;241:24171–9.
19. van Veenendaal N, Poelman M, Apers J, Cense H, Schreurs H, Sonneveld E, et al. The INCH-trial: a multicenter randomized controlled trial comparing short- and long-term outcomes of open and laparoscopic surgery for incisional hernia repair. Surg Endosc. 2023;37(12):9147–58.
20. Fields AC, Gonzalez DO, Chin EH, Nguyen SQ, Zhang LP, Divino CM. Laparoscopic-assisted transversus abdominis plane block for postoperative pain control in laparoscopic ventral hernia repair: a randomized controlled trial. J Am Coll Surg. 2015;221(2):462–9.
21. Paasch C, Santo G, Aljedani N, Ortiz P, Bruckert L, Hünerbein M, Lorenz E, Croner R. The effect of an abdominal binder on postoperative pain after laparoscopic incisional hernia repair– a multicenter, randomized pilot trial (ABIHR-I) of the intraperitoneal Onlay-mesh technique. Dtsch Arztebl Int. 2021;118(37):607–13. https://doi.org/10.3238/arztebl.m2021.0250. Epub 2021 Sep 24. PMID: 34857076; PMCID: PMC8704821
22. Khan S, Siddiqa M, Rehman HU. Comparison of frequency of seroma formation in laparoscopic para umbilical hernia repair with and without primary closure of defect. J Pak Med Assoc. 2022;72(2):265–9.
23. Christoffersen MW, Westen M, Rosenberg J, Helgstrand F, Bisgaard T. Closure of the fascial defect during laparoscopic umbilical hernia repair: a randomized clinical trial. Br J Surg. 2020;107(3):200–8.
24. LeBlanc K. Proper mesh overlap is a key determinant in hernia recurrence following laparoscopic ventral and incisional hernia repair. Hernia. 2016;20(1):85–99.

Chapter 13
Laparoscopic Parastomal Hernia Repair

Emeka Ray-Offor, Emanuele Lo Menzo, Samuel Szomstein, and Raul J. Rosenthal

E. Ray-Offor (✉)
College of Health Sciences, University of Port Harcourt, Choba, Rivers State, Nigeria

Colorectal/Minimal Access Surgery Unit, Department of Surgery, University of Port Harcourt Teaching Hospital, Port Harcourt, Rivers State, Nigeria
e-mail: emeka.ray-offor@uniport.edu.ng

E. L. Menzo
Department of General Surgery, Program Cleveland Clinic Florida, The Bariatric and Metabolic Institute, Ellen Leifer Shulman and Steven Shulman Digestive Disease Center, Weston, FL, USA

Charles E. Schmidt College of Medicine, Florida Atlantic University, Boca Raton, FL, USA

Herbert Wertheim College of Medicine, Florida International University, Miami, FL, USA

S. Szomstein
Department of General Surgery, The Bariatric and Metabolic Institute, Ellen Leifer Shulman and Steven Shulman Digestive Disease Center, Cleveland Clinic Florida, Weston, FL, USA

Herbert Wertheim College of Medicine, Florida International University, Miami, FL, USA

R. J. Rosenthal
The Bariatric and Metabolic Institute, Ellen Leifer Shulman and Steven Shulman Digestive Disease Center, Cleveland Clinic Florida, Weston, FL, USA

Cleveland Clinic Lerner College of Medicine at Case Western Reserve University, Cleveland, OH, USA

Charles E. Schmidt College of Medicine, Florida Atlantic University, Boca Raton, FL, USA

Herbert Wertheim College of Medicine, Florida International University, Miami, FL, USA

Introduction

Parastomal hernias (PSHs) are fascial defects adjacent to the stoma site following ileostomy and colostomy operations [1]. They are separately classified incisional hernias and the most frequent complication of end colostomy [2]. In comparison to the other types of stoma creation, PSHs are more common with end colostomy and incidence increases over time, with a range from 3% to 48%, and up to almost 30% after ileostomy creation [3, 4]. As life expectancy after cancer treatment rises with more surgeries performed, the incidence of PSH is also expected to rise. More frequent etiologic factors are patient related and include obesity, wound infections, steroid use, malnutrition, old age, and increased intra-abdominal pressure [5]. Other aetiologic factors include surgeon related factors like diameter of the trephine, whether the stoma is constructed in an emergency setting and whether an intraperitoneal or extraperitoneal approach is used [6].

Asymptomatic PSHs can be managed conservatively with weight loss, patient education, and an ostomy hernia belt; however, an estimated 30–56% of the patients with PSH will ultimately require surgical repair [7]. The options for surgical repair include stoma relocation, fascial suture, and mesh repair. Mesh repair is associated with relatively lower risk of recurrence than the other two options [8]. Following the success of laparoscopic mesh repair for ventral hernia with the benefits for patients including quicker recovery and lower postoperative pain, a laparoscopic approach to repair has been extended to PSHs. Laparoscopic approach to repair has the unique advantage of visualization of the entire anterior abdominal wall to detect any non-palpable hernia which can be concurrently repaired. Laparoscopic repair of parastomal hernias theoretically provides an excellent anatomic correction of such defects. Adhesions are lysed under magnified laparoscopic vision, and the true limits of the fascial defects are clearly identified.

The two major surgical techniques used laparoscopically for repair of PSH are the keyhole and modified Sugarbaker techniques [9, 10]. While both techniques involve an intraperitoneal placement of mesh, the difference being that bowel is exteriorized through the side of the mesh in the modified Sugarbaker approach whereas the bowel is inserted through a 2–3 cm slit in the center of the mesh for the keyhole approach. Sugarbaker repairs for parastomal hernia are significantly less often associated with recurrence when compared to keyhole repairs [11, 12]. A prophylactic mesh placement at the time of stoma creation is known to reduce the rate of parastomal hernia, without an increase in mesh-related complications [13].

Relevant Anatomy

The anterior abdominal wall encloses the anterior lateral aspect of the abdominal cavity. It comprises skin, subcutaneous tissue (with blood vessels and nerves), muscles, fascia, and parietal peritoneum. The five muscles in the abdominal wall are

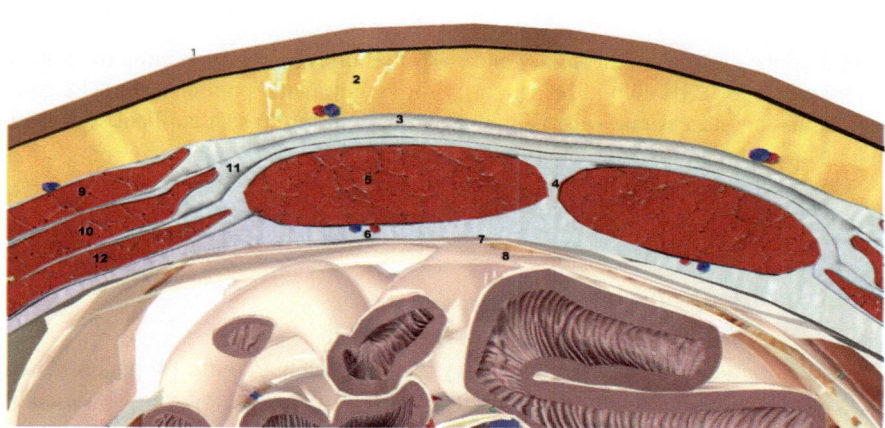

Fig. 13.1 Axial section of anterior abdominal wall below the arcuate line: (1) Skin; (2) Subcutaneous layer; (3) Anterior rectus sheath; (4) Linea alba; (5) Rectus abdominis muscle; (6) Inferior epigastric vessels; (7)Transversalis fascia; (8) Peritoneum; (9)External oblique muscle; (10) Internal oblique muscle; (11) Aponeurosis; (12) Transversus abdominis muscle. (Adapted from Anterior abdominal wall www.shutterstock.com)

divided into two groups (vertical and flat) with an aponeurosis formed by these muscles (rectus sheath) [14]. The two vertical muscles are situated near the midline of the body (rectus abdominis) and the three flat muscles are located laterally and stacked on top of each other (Fig. 13.1). The three flat muscles include the external oblique, internal oblique, and transversus abdominis. The rectus sheath is a condensation of the aponeurosis of these flat muscles with the anterior rectus sheath formed by contribution from the external oblique and half of the internal oblique. The posterior rectus sheath is formed by the inner half of the aponeurosis of the internal oblique and that from transversus abdominis. Midway between the umbilicus and pubic symphysis, the posterior rectus disappears at the arcuate line. Distal to this point the rectus muscle is in direct apposition with the underlying transversalis fascia.

PSH is an abnormal protrusion of the contents of the abdominal cavity through the abdominal wall defect created during the placement of a colostomy, ileostomy, or ileal conduit stoma [15]. Peritoneal sac contents of the hernia may include omentum, small bowel, stomach, and colon.

There are different classification systems for parastomal hernias that are based on size, location, contents, and radiologic findings associated with the hernia. A subgroup classification of PSH by Delvin and Rubin into four types of parastomal hernias comprises: Interstitial; Subcutaneous; Intrastomal and Peristomal [16]. The European Hernia Society classification of parastomal hernias has four types based on the PSH defect size with small as ≤5 cm and the presence of a concomitant incisional hernia (cIH) This comprises: small PSH without cIH (Type I); small PH with cIH (Type II); large PH without cIH (Type III); and large PH with cIH (Type IV) [17].

Indications

Based on the significant morbidity and risk of recurrence, the indication of surgical intervention for PSH should be primarily for symptomatic patients [18]. The complications that necessitate surgery include pain, inability to seal appliances, intestinal obstruction, and strangulation [19].

Cosmesis is yet another indication for surgery.

Contraindications

Generally, patients with cardiopulmonary disorders who are unfit for general anesthesia or with coagulation disorder are unsuitable for laparoscopic surgery. Specific contraindications to laparoscopic parastomal hernia repair are patients with identified tumor recurrence or having uncontrolled infections of the urinary tract, lung, or skin near the stoma [20].

Preoperative Preparation

It is pertinent to distinguish PSH from local stoma problems without a hernia sac, such as a mucosal prolapse or a subcutaneous folding of the excess bowel length at the stoma. A full clinical and radiological assessment of the patient is needed with the identification of other anterior abdominal wall hernias and comorbidities for an adequate workup for surgery.

The OR equipment comprise a laparoscopy set, trocars (one 10–12 mm and two 5 mm), suction/irrigation device, atraumatic graspers, dissecting scissors, suture passer, and mesh fixator (e.g. Pro Tack Covidien). Energy appliances can be diathermy with L-hook electrode or a Harmonic generator with laparoscopic shears or other suitable devices. Ideally a composite mesh made up of a permanent synthetic material for the parietal side to encourage adhesion formation and an adhesion barrier layer for contact with the visceral side is recommended [21]. The application of a non-protected polypropylene mesh intraperitoneally is discouraged as it harbours the risk for extensive adhesions, bowel fistula and mesh infection [22]. Size of the mesh should be large enough to ensure an overlap of the mesh beyond the hernia defect in all directions of at least 5 cm.

A limited bowel preparation can be administered but prophylactic broad spectrum intravenous antibiotics in the immediate preoperative period is mandatory.

Technique

General anaesthesia is administered. Patient is in supine and Trendelenburg position on the operating table. A routine cleaning of operating field with povidone iodine is made with emphasis on the peristomal area. A catheter is inserted into the stoma for ease of intraoperative identification of stoma limb and the stoma then isolated from the operative field using adhesive transparent film dressing.

A 12 mm camera trocar is placed under direct vision at the right flank to avoid adhesions from previous possible midline surgery. Capnoperitoneum is achieved at 12–15 mmHg. Two 5 mm working trocars are placed at the right and left lower abdomen. Following laparoscopic entry, a diagnostic exploration is made then adequate adhesiolysis and careful reduction of hernia sac contents are performed. A combination of external hand pressure and intraabdominal traction with atraumatic forceps are applied for reduction of sac content. The adhesions are separated by sharp scissors dissection or an appropriate energy device. Great care is taken to avoid injury to bowel; a tug on the catheter inserted into the stoma at onset of surgery aids identification of stoma limb of bowel in adhesion. The fascial defect must be clearly seen by the end of hernia sac content reduction (Fig. 13.2).

A tape is inserted into the 12 mm trocar an accurate measurement of the defect is made with the capnoperitoneum temporarily reduced to 8 mmHg. Using 2–0 Prolene suture the bowel is lateralized by applying two anchor stitches to the serosa of stoma bowel at two fixed opposite sides to the parietal peritoneum just lateral to the defect. A large defect is repaired using an intracorporeal continuous shoelace technique with a single non-absorbable suture before an intraperitoneal onlay mesh placement (Fig. 13.3). Alternatively, a barbed suture may be used [23].

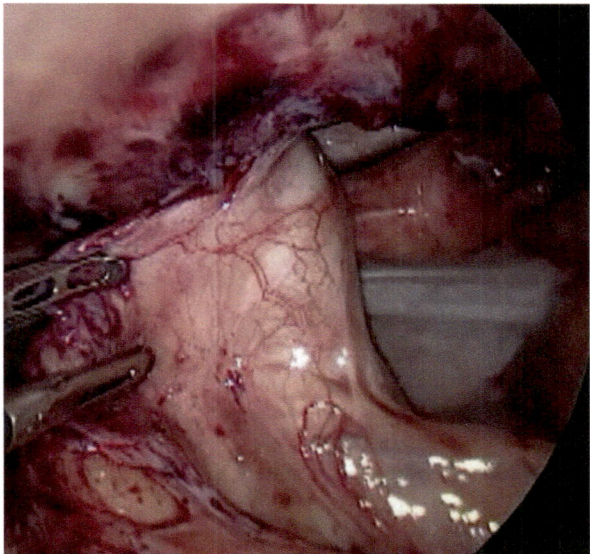

Fig. 13.2 Parastomal defect after dissection

Fig. 13.3 Sutured parastomal defect

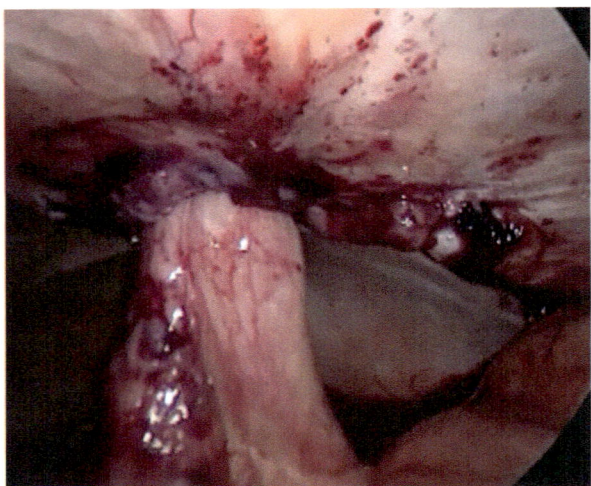

Fig. 13.4 Placement and orientation of mesh

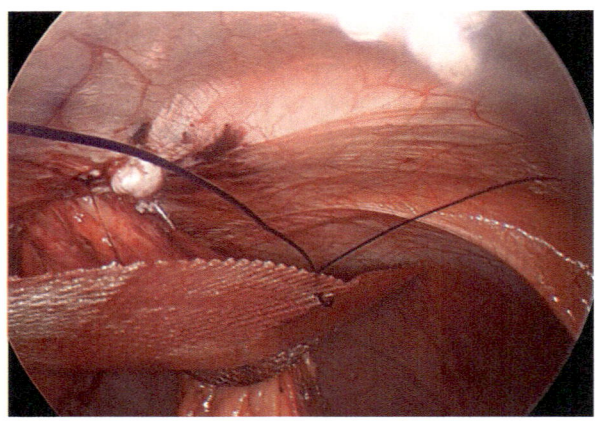

The composite mesh is prepared with an overlap of 5 cm on all sides of the defect. For a rectangular mesh, a 2.0 Prolene suture is used to apply 4 knots to each of the angles of the mesh with a long tail end and the needle end of the suture cut to the same distance. The mesh is rolled around the long shaft of laparoscopic forceps, internalizing the sutures applied on the synthetic side of mesh and then introduce peritoneally via the 12 mm trocar. A tiny stab incision is made on the anterior abdominal wall skin starting over the superior lateral angle of the mesh overlap. Through the incision, a suture passer delivers externally both ends of the suture sequentially which are grasped with forceps. A similar procedure is performed for the other 3 sites (Fig. 13.4).

In like manner, the other superior angle followed by the lower ones are secured. Fastening transfascial knots are then made after checking the correctness of the mesh position and the knot buried in the stab incisions. Using a Pro tack mesh

Fig. 13.5 Mesh reinforcement with double row of spiral tackers

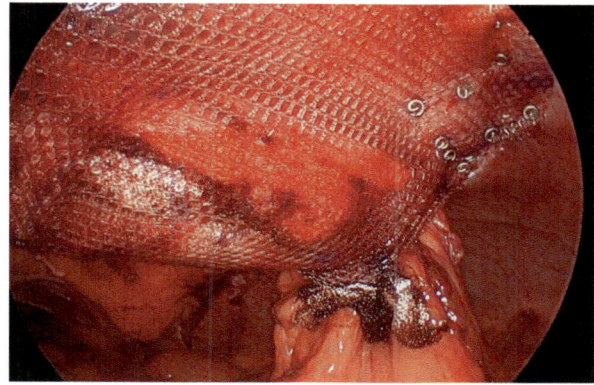

fixator an inner crown of tacks is applied along the margin of the defect and on either side of the lateralized bowel avoiding bowel injury. An external crown of tacks is then applied to all edges of the mesh except the area overhanging the lateralized limb. A reasonable amount of space is left to accommodate the passage of stool through the lateralized bowel (Fig. 13.5).

Following this, a final inspection for hemostasis is made, the capnoperitoneum is released completely, and fascia closure of the 10 mm port is done, and a dressing is applied. Film dressing occluding stoma is removed. Skin strips are applied to the stab wounds.

Post-operative Care

The postoperative care of patients after parastomal hernia repair is as previously discussed for incisional hernia repair in Chap. 12. Generally, abdominal binders are applied for 4–6 weeks to reduce seroma complications. During this period, the patient is encouraged not to lift heavy objects and to avoid strenuous activity. Recurrence is a long-term complication associated with parastomal hernia repair.

References

1. Pilgrim CH, McIntyre R, Bailey M. Prospective audit of parastomal hernia: prevalence and associated comorbidities. Dis Colon Rectum. 2010;53:71–7.
2. Antoniou SA, Agresta F, Garcia Alamino JM, Berger D, Berrevoet F, Brandsma HT, et al. European hernia society guidelines on prevention and treatment of parastomal hernias. Hernia. 2018;22:183–98.
3. Rubin MS, Schoetz DJ Jr, Matthews JB. Parastomal hernia. Is stoma relocation superior to fascial repair? Arch Surg. 1994;129:413e418.

4. Antoniou SA, Agresta F, Garcia Alamino JM, et al. European hernia society guidelines on prevention and treatment of parastomal hernias. Hernia. 2018;22(1):183–98.
5. Nastro P, Knowles CH, McGrath A. Complications of intestinal stomas. Br J Surg. 2010;97:1885–9.
6. Carne PW, Robertson GM, Frizelle FA. Parastomal hernia. Br J Surg. 2003;90(7):784–93.
7. Ripoche J, Basurko C, Fabbro-Perray P, Prudhomme M, Parastomal hernia. A study of the French federation of ostomy patients. J Vis Surg. 2011;148(6):e435–41.
8. Slater NJ, Hansson BM, Buyne OR. Repair of parastomal hernias with biologic grafts a systematic review. J Gastrointest Surg. 2011;15:1252–8.
9. Shah NR, Craft RO, Harold KL. Parastomal hernia repair. Surg Clin North Am. 2013;93:1185–98.
10. Hotouras A, Murphy J, Thaha M, Chan CL. The persistent challenge of parastomal herniation: a review of the literature and future developments. Color Dis. 2013;15:e202–14.
11. DeAsis FJ, Lapin B, Gitelis ME, Ujiki MB. Current state of laparoscopic parastomal hernia repair: a meta-analysis. World J Gastroenterol. 2015;21(28):8670–7.
12. Fleming AM, Phillips AL, Drake JA, Gross MG, Yakoub D, Monroe J, et al. Sugarbaker versus keyhole repair for parastomal hernia: a systematic review and meta-analysis of comparative studies. J Gastrointest Surg. 2023;27:573–84.
13. Cross AJ, Buchwald PL, Frizelle FA, Eglinton TW. Meta-analysis of prophylactic mesh to prevent parastomal hernia. Br J Surg. 2017;104(3):179–86. https://doi.org/10.1002/bjs.10402. Epub 2016 Dec 22
14. Varacallo M, Scharbach S, Al-Dhahir MA. Anatomy, anterolateral abdominal wall muscles. [Updated 2023 Jul 24]. In: StatPearls [Internet]. Treasure Island, FL: StatPearls Publishing; 2023. https://www.ncbi.nlm.nih.gov/books/NBK470334/.
15. Muysoms F, Campanelli G, Champault GG. EuraHS: the development of an international online platform for registration and outcome measurement of ventral abdominal wall hernia repair. Hernia. 2012;16:239–50.
16. Devlin HB, Kingsnorth AN. Management of abdominal wall hernias. 2nd ed. London: Chapman & Hall; 1998. p. 39–41.
17. Śmietański M, Szczepkowski M, Alexandre JA, Berger D, Bury K, Conze J, Hansson B, Janes A, Miserez M, Mandala V, Montgomery A, Morales Conde S, Muysoms F. European hernia society classification of parastomal hernias. Hernia. 2014 Feb;18(1):1–6.
18. Tivenius M, Nasvall P, Sandblom G. Parastomal hernias causing symptoms or requiring surgical repair after colorectal cancer surgery-a national population-based cohort study. Int J Color Dis. 2019;34(7):1267–72.
19. Tsujinaka S, Tan KY, Miyakura Y, Fukano R, Oshima M, Konishi F, Rikiyama T. Current management of intestinal stomas and their complications. J Anus Rectum Colon. 2020;4(1):25–33.
20. Yang X, He K, Hua R, Shen Q, Yao Q. Laparoscopic repair of parastomal hernia. Ann Transl Med. 2017;5(3):45.
21. Deeken CR, Faucher KM, Matthews BD. A review of the composition, characteristics, and effectiveness of barrier mesh prostheses utilized for laparoscopic ventral hernia repair. Surg Endosc. 2012;26(2):566–7.
22. Mancini GJ, Mcclusky DA 3rd, Khaitan L, Goldenberg EA, Heniford BT, Novitsky YW, et al. Laparoscopic parastomal hernia repair using a non-slit mesh technique. Surg Endosc. 2007;21:1487–91.
23. Silva E, Szomstein S, Van Koughnett JA, Rosenthal R, Wexner S. A new combined technique of reinforced parastomal hernia repair. J Am Coll Surg. 2014;219(5):e55–7.

Chapter 14
Transabdominal Preperitoneal Hernia Repair (TAPP)

Usman Mohammed Bello

Historical Perspective

Laparoscopic hernia repair involves reinforcement of the transversalis fascia in the myopectineal orifice as earlier described by Rives and Stoppa [1]. Ger in 1982 first attempted indirect inguinal hernia repair by closing the internal ring with metal clips [2]. The first laparoscopic repair of groin hernia is credited to Pletcher in 1979 [3]. Since then several surgeons have described similar repairs with their outcomes [4–8]. In 1991, intraperitoneal onlay mesh placement to cover the internal ring was described by Toy and Smoot [9]. Due to the observed adhesions because of the abdominal entry in trans abdominal preperitoneal hernia repair (TAPP), Dulucq Jan Louis developed Totally Extraperitoneal Hernia repair (TEP) [10]. This involves dissection in the preperitoneal space, thus avoiding intra-abdominal dissection with consequent adhesions. This approach, however, is more difficult due to narrow space, especially in obese patients. It also has a steep learning curve. Jorge Daes in 1999 is credited with the development of Extended View totally extraperitoneal hernia repair (E-TEP). This is to circumvent the difficulties of TEP as it provides a wider surgical field in the extraperitoneal space [11]. This technique is now used to repair all hernias including ventral and incisional hernia using the extraperitoneal space. Igor Belyansky and Yuri Novitsky modified the above-mentioned technique in ventral hernia surgery [12].

U. M. Bello (✉)
Aminu Kano Teaching Hospital, Kano, Kano State, Nigeria

Bayero University, Kano, Kano State, Nigeria

Relevant Anatomy

As in open inguinal hernia surgery, a good knowledge of anatomy is critical. It is important to know the anatomy of the lower anterior abdominal wall as viewed from inside during laparoscopy (Fig. 14.1). There are important landmarks that need to be identified. These are important double folds of the parietal peritoneum (ligaments) and certain triangles formed by the structures in this region.

The ligaments include:

1. Median umbilical ligament: This ligament is the obliterated urachus and extends from the dome of the urinary bladder to the umbilicus.
2. Medial umbilical ligaments: These are the paired ligaments located on either side of the midline. They are the most prominent and represent obliterated umbilical artery (Fig. 14.2). They are the medial limit of the peritoneal incision to gain access to the retroperitoneal space at the beginning of the surgery when raising the peritoneal flap.
3. Lateral umbilical Ligaments: These are less prominent than the medial umbilical ligament and contain the inferior epigastric vessels.

An important landmark is the inverted Y sign (Fig. 14.3). This is formed by the inferior epigastric vessels above and inferiorly the limbs are formed by the vas deferens inferior medially and the gonadal vessels inferior laterally. A horizontal line passing at the midpoint of the limbs (which corresponds to the internal ring) forms 3 triangles below the line. The lateral triangle formed by the transverse imaginary

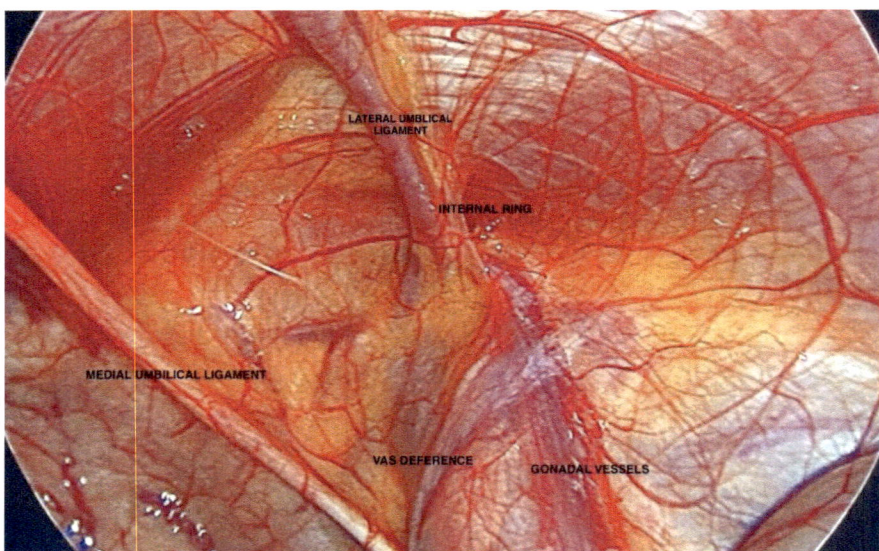

Fig. 14.1 Laparoscopic view of right myopectineal orifice demonstrating hernial orifices and important structures

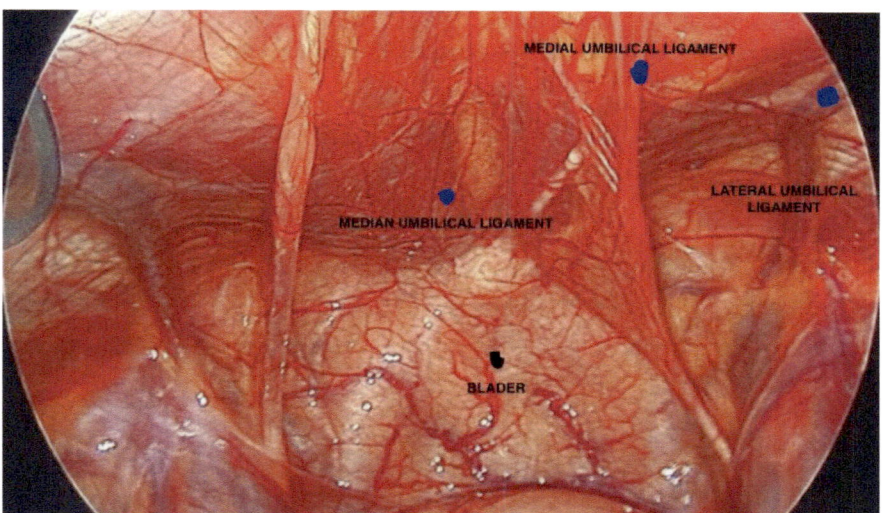

Fig. 14.2 Laparoscopic view of anterior abdominal wall

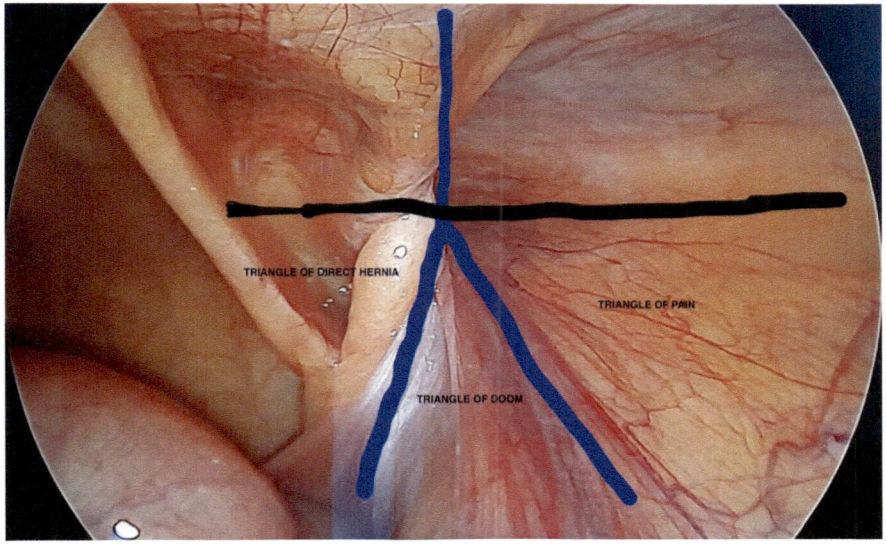

Fig. 14.3 Laparoscopic view showing the triangles. (Inverted Y in blue)

line and the inferior lateral limb which corresponds with the gonadal vessels is called the Triangle of Pain. It is referred to this way because the important sensory nerves are located within it, viz., ilioinguinal nerve, genitofemoral nerve, and lateral femoral cutaneous nerve of the thigh. The middle triangle is the triangle of death or the Triangle of Doom. The contents are the external iliac artery and vein. Injury to any of these structures can be catastrophic. The medial is the Triangle of Direct hernia (Fig. 14.4). An indirect hernia arises lateral to the lateral umbilical ligament (Figs. 14.5 and 14.6).

Indications

Laparoscopic hernia surgery has become well established, with increasing boundaries, especially in ventral hernia repair. The indications for TAPP are as follows:

1. *Bilateral Hernia:* In bilateral groin hernia the advantage is that both hernias can be repaired with two 5 mm ports, thus avoiding the trauma of bilateral groin incision.
2. *Recurrent inguinal hernia:* Because of the previous surgery, the inguinal canal anatomy is distorted, this makes redo operation through the same space more prone to injury to vas deferens, testicular vessels, and occasionally bowel and bladder injury.
3. *Unilateral Hernia:* Recent studies have shown superior benefits of laparoscopic transabdominal preperitoneal hernia repair in terms of less pain and early return to work even for unilateral hernia compared to open surgery.
4. *Concomitant Unilateral Hernia and other intraabdominal conditions:* Examples include inguinal hernia coexisting with symptomatic adhesions, or other intra-abdominal conditions requiring concomitant laparoscopic treatment.

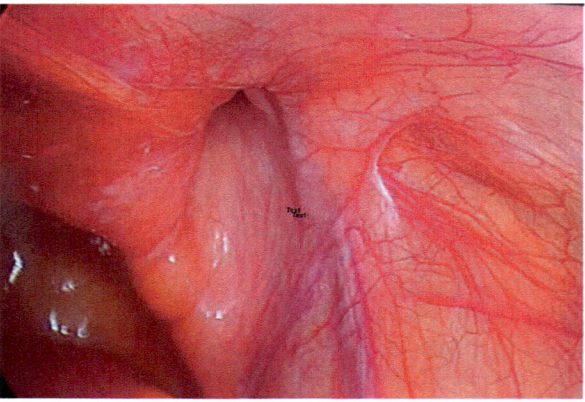

Fig. 14.4 Anatomy of the right inguinal region at laparoscopy with indirect and direct hernia openings

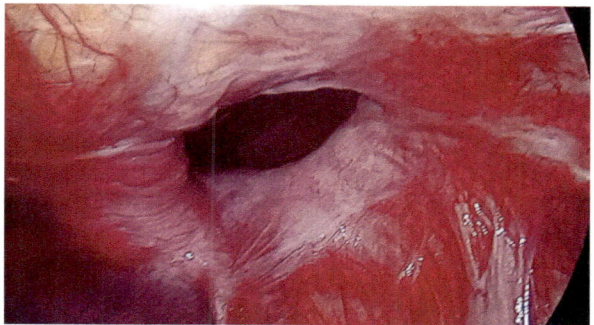

Fig. 14.5 Indirect Inguinal hernia with wide defect as viewed at laparoscopy

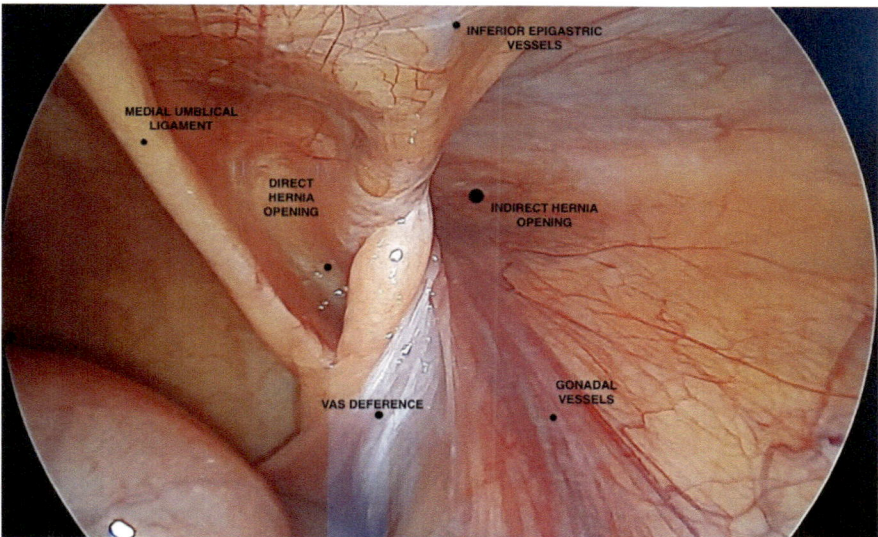

Fig. 14.6 Direct and Indirect inguinal hernias

Contraindications

These are mainly complicated hernias where the surgery may be difficult or pose the possibility of complications such as bowel injury. Some of these however are presently relative contraindications as indicated in the bracket. This is due to improvement in laparoscopic surgical skills and improved laparoscopic instrumentation:

1. Giant inguinoscrotal hernia (**Relative**)
2. Incarcerated inguinal hernia (**Relative**)
3. Prior retroperitoneal pelvic surgery i.e., pelvic lymph node dissection, radical prostatectomy (**Relative**)
4. Prior pelvic irradiation.
5. Infraumbilical laparotomies or previous attempts of TAPP.

6. Cardiopulmonary disease contraindicating general anesthesia.
7. Coagulopathy

Preoperative Preparation

Laparoscopic groin hernia surgery is done under general anesthesia with muscle relaxation; hence patients need to be fully evaluated to determine fitness for undergoing general anesthesia. Investigations such as echocardiogram, electrocardiogram (ECG), and spirometry may be needed to rule out cardiac disease and chronic obstructive pulmonary disease (COPD). Other investigations needed include complete blood count, electrolytes, urea, and creatinine level.

A laparoscopic system with high definition (HD) imaging is preferable with a 30-degree telescope which is better for visualizing pelvic cavity and anterior abdominal wall during upper dissection. Two standard graspers, polypropylene mesh of 15 by 15 cm in size which is trimmed to 15 by 10 cm are essential. There are however 3D meshes that are shaped to fit in the preperitoneal space with ease of placement. A mesh fixation device is also needed to keep the mesh in position to prevent rolling after desufflation. The most used is the tacker which has clips that fix the mesh. Tackers can be absorbable or non-absorbable. Other items needed include scissors, needle holders, and energy devices for hemostasis.

Anesthesia

General anesthesia with muscle relaxation is the mainstay. There is also a need for monitoring of cardiopulmonary vital signs such as pulse and respiratory rate, blood pressure, ECG, pulse oximetry, and end-tidal carbon dioxide levels.

Positioning

The patient will be in a supine position with the foot of the bed raised to a 15-degree position to allow the bowel to fall back and aid its reduction into the abdomen. A urethral catheter is also passed for bladder decompression. The surgeon stands on the side opposite the hernia while the camera assistant can stand on the same side or opposite to the surgeon. In bilateral hernia, the team moves to the opposite side to operate on the contralateral hernia.

Access and Trocar Placement

Closed or open access technique is done, and the abdomen is insufflated with carbon dioxide CO_2 to a pressure of 12–15 mmHg. The optical trocar is inserted at the umbilicus; two other 5 mm working ports are inserted on a horizontal line 10 cm from the umbilicus (Fig. 14.7). The working port on the side of the hernia however is placed about 2 finger breaths above the horizontal line for better ergonomics. In bilateral hernia repair, trocars can be placed at the same level. Diagnostic laparoscopy is first done to check for adhesions and other intra-abdominal pathology. The hernia contents are normally reduced after insufflation, if there are no adhesions between the contents and the peritoneum. Sometimes, adhesiolysis may have to be done to reduce the contents. The hernia opening usually becomes obvious after the contents are reduced. In the case of indirect hernia, it is seen lateral to the inferior epigastric artery, while direct is medial to it.

Technique

The procedure begins with a peritoneal incision 3–4 cm above the internal ring. The incision is extended laterally to reach 2-finger breath medial to anterior superior iliac supine which is determined by finger pressure from outside the abdomen by the surgeon or assistant. Medially, it is extended to the medial umbilical ligament. This incision can be done with cold scissors, electrocautery, or harmonic scalpel. The preperitoneal pocket is then developed starting laterally in the space of Bogros (Triangle of pain), then medially. The dissection medially is done to the pubic bone where the iliopubic tract is seen. The dissection is also carried to about 2 cm below the pubic bone to allow for proper placement of the mesh and allows the mesh to cover the femoral opening thus preventing the development of a femoral hernia.

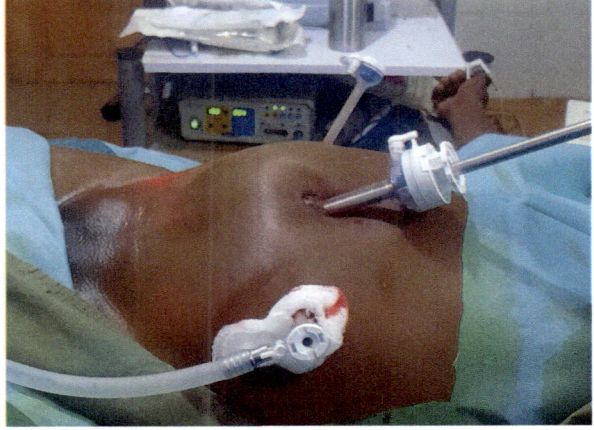

Fig. 14.7 Port placement during right inguinal herniorrhaphy

During this pelvic dissection, care must be taken concerning corona mortis veins which can bleed excessively when injured. The lower extent of dissection is where the vas deferens crosses the iliac vessels turning medially towards the bladder. The last part is the dissection of the sac from the cord structures. This is done by gently stripping it from the vas deferens and the gonadal vessels. In the inguinoscrotal hernia where the sac extends into the scrotum, the sac can be divided in the middle. Special care must be taken in dissection in the Triangle of Doom to avoid injuries to iliac vessels.

After creating the preperitoneal pocket, the 10 by 15 cm polypropylene mesh is placed via the umbilical port after rolling it. Where available 3D mesh, which is shaped to fit into the preperitoneal space can be placed. Various mesh fixation devices are used to fix the mesh; these include fibrin glue and Tackers (absorbable and non-absorbable). The author commonly uses an absorbable tacker (Fig. 14.8).

After the mesh placement and fixation (Fig. 14.9), the peritoneal flap is closed to cover the mesh (Fig. 14.10). This helps to prevent adhesion formation and fistulation between the mesh and the bowel. This closure can be achieved by Tackers or intracorporeal suture. If there are inadvertent holes in the peritoneum during the dissection, they need to be closed to avoid mesh exposure, with consequent adhesions. The abdomen is desufflated and the ports are subsequently closed in layers. In 10 and 12 mm ports, the fascia is closed with non-absorbable suture, after which a subcuticular skin closure is done as there is about 2% chance of hernia if the fascia is not closed; while for 5 mm ports, only the skin is closed.

Fig. 14.8 Hernia Tacker

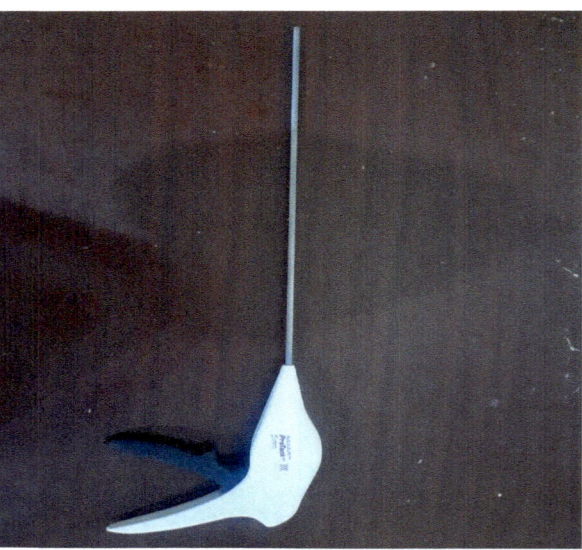

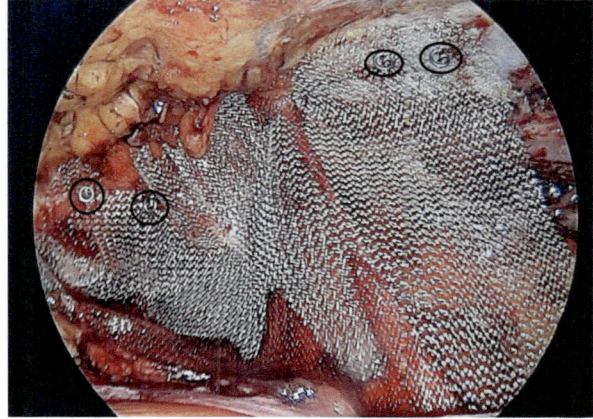

Fig. 14.9 Laparoscopic view of polypropylene mesh in the dissected right myopectineal orifice fixed with tacker pins (rounded in black circles)

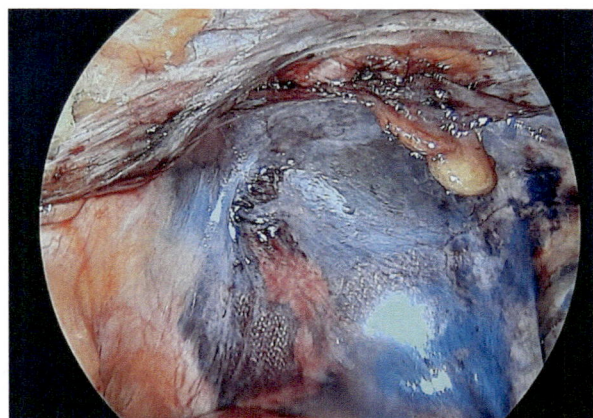

Fig. 14.10 Mesh covered with peritoneal flap

Complications

Anesthesia-Related

Since general anesthesia is needed for the surgery, complications related to this may occasionally be seen (Refer to the chapter on Anesthesia in Principles and Practice of Laparoscopic Surgery Volume I).

Access Related

These include:

1. Vascular injuries (inferior epigastric, aortic, and common iliac artery injury)
2. Bowel injury
3. Port site infection
4. Port site hernia

Pneumoperitoneum Related

1. Hypotension
2. Gas embolism
3. Cardiac arrest

Surgery Related

1. Injury to cord structures
2. Vascular injuries (external iliac artery or vein, inferior epigastric vessels, and corona mortis)
3. Nerve injury (lateral femoral cutaneous nerve of the thigh, Genito femoral nerve, and ilioinguinal nerve)
4. Adhesions and adhesive intestinal obstruction
5. Recurrence

Challenges of Laparoscopic Hernia Surgery in Low- and Middle-income Countries

Laparoscopic surgery is quite expensive due to the need to procure expensive equipment, the need for expensive consumables, and training. This is particularly so while moving to advanced laparoscopic surgery. In low- and middle-income countries budgetary allocation to health is poor and the healthcare focus is mainly in areas of tackling infections and other primary healthcare challenges. Insurance where available is limited to an insignificant percentage of the population and most times does not cover most laparoscopic procedures. So, most patients pay out of pocket despite low per capita income.

An important area of circumventing cost is the use of reusable instruments where possible instead of disposable consumables, this will help share the cost among some patients. Laparoscopic surgery though incorporated in the National Health insurance scheme, is limited to basic procedures and not appropriately priced. So, incorporating other advanced procedures with appropriate pricing to cover all consumables will go a long way in increasing access by patients.

References

1. Stoppa RE, Rives JL, Warlaumont CR, Palot JP, Verhaeghe PJ, Delattre JF. The use of Dacron in the repair of hernias of the groin. Surg Clin North Am. 1984;64:269–85.
2. Mishra RK. Textbook of practical laparoscopic surgery. 3rd ed. New Delhi: Jaypee Brothers Medical Publishers; 2013.
3. Read RC. Milestones in the history of hernia surgery: prosthetic repair. Hernia. 2004;8:8–14.
4. Ger R. The management of certain abdominal herniae by intra-abdominal closure of the neck of the sac. Preliminary communication. Ann R Coll Surg Engl. 1982;64:342–4.
5. Bogojavlensky S, editor Laparoscopic treatment of inguinal and femoral hernias. Proceedings of the 18th Annual meeting of the American Association of Gynecological Laparoscopists, Washington, DC; 1989.
6. Schultz L, Graber J, Pietrafitta J, Hickok D. Laser laparoscopic herniorraphy: a clinical trial preliminary result. J Laparoendosc Surg. 1990;1:41–5.
7. Arregui ME, Navarrete J, Davis CJ, Castro D, Nagan RF. Laparoscopic inguinal herniorrhaphy. Techniques and controversies. Surg Clin North Am. 1993;73:513–27.
8. Arregui ME, Davis CJ, Yucel O, Nagan RF. Laparoscopic mesh repair of inguinal hernia using a preperitoneal approach: a preliminary report. Surg Laparosc Endosc. 1992;2:53–8.
9. Toy FK, Smoot RT Jr. Toy-smooth laparoscopic hernioplasty. Surg Laparosc Endosc. 1991;1:151–5.
10. Dulucq J. Traitement des hernies de l'aine par la mise en place d'un patch prothetique par laparoscopie. Voi totalement extraperitoneale. Cah Chir. 1991;79:15–6.
11. Daes J. Reparo laparoscopico de lahernia inguinal. Experiencia de la Unidad de laparoscopia. Clinica Bautista, Barranquilla. Rev Colomb Cir. 1999;14:97–103.
12. Belyansky I, Daes J, Radu VG, Balasubramanian R, Reza Zahiri H, Weltz AS, et al. A novel approach using the enhanced view totally extraperitoneal (eTEP) technique for laparoscopic retromuscular hernia repair. Surg Endosc. 2018;32:1525–32.

Chapter 15
Totally Extraperitoneal Hernia Repair

Yin Min Benjamin Tan, Samuel Szomstein, Emanuele Lo Menzo, and Raul J. Rosenthal

Y. M. B. Tan (✉)
General, Minimally Invasive and Bariatric Surgery, Cleveland Clinic Florida, Weston, FL, USA

S. Szomstein
Ellen Leifer Shulman, and Steven Shulman Digestive Disease Center, Cleveland Clinic Florida, Weston, FL, USA

Florida International University, Miami, FL, USA

E. L. Menzo
Department of General Surgery, Program Cleveland Clinic Florida, The Bariatric and Metabolic Institute, Ellen Leifer Shulman and Steven Shulman Digestive Disease Center, Weston, FL, USA

Charles E. Schmidt College of Medicine, Florida Atlantic University, Boca Raton, FL, USA

Florida International University College of Medicine, Miami, FL, USA

R. J. Rosenthal
Ellen Leifer Shulman and Steven Shulman Digestive Disease Institute, Cleveland Clinic Florida, Weston, FL, USA

Division of General Surgery, Cleveland Clinic Florida, Weston, FL, USA

Cleveland Clinic Lerner College of Medicine at Case Western Reserve University, Cleveland, OH, USA

Charles E. Schmidt College of Medicine, Florida Atlantic University, Boca Raton, FL, USA

Herbert Wertheim College of Medicine, Florida International University, Miami, FL, USA

© The Author(s), under exclusive license to Springer Nature Switzerland AG 2024
E. Ray-Offor, R. J. Rosenthal (eds.), *Colorectal & Hernia Laparoscopic Surgery*, https://doi.org/10.1007/978-3-031-63490-1_15

Historical Perspective

Inguinal hernias have been known and treated for centuries. The first recorded attempts at hernia repair date back to ancient Egypt around 1500 BCE [1]. Throughout history, various surgical techniques have been developed to repair inguinal hernias, with varying degrees of success. The modern era of inguinal hernia repair began in the nineteenth century with the introduction of tension repair techniques. These techniques involved suturing the edges of the hernia defect to strengthen the weakened abdominal wall. However, these methods often resulted in a high rate of recurrence and complications. In the late twentieth century, laparoscopic techniques revolutionized hernia surgery. Laparoscopic inguinal hernia repair, including the totally extraperitoneal (TEP) approach, emerged as a minimally invasive alternative to open surgery. The TEP technique was first described by McKernan and Laws in 1993 and gained popularity in the following years [2].

An inguinal hernia occurs when there is a defect in the tissue of the inguinal region. An indirect inguinal hernia occurs when there is a defect through the internal inguinal ring and protrusion of the hernia into the inguinal canal. This occurs lateral to the inferior epigastric vessels [3]. In a direct inguinal hernia, the defect is at the floor of the inguinal canal medial to the inferior epigastric vessels, through a weakened transversalis fascia. A femoral hernia is through a defect of the femoral canal, inferior to the inguinal ligament and medial to the femoral vein. Laparoscopic Totally Extra-Peritoneal repair (TEP) repair is a safe and effective alternative to the traditional open hernia repair and is performed using small incisions and a camera to visualize the hernia and repair it from within the extra-peritoneal layer. The hernia is repaired by placing a mesh patch over the weak area of the myopectineal orifice, reinforcing it and preventing further protrusion of the intestine or herniated contents. The benefits of Laparoscopic TEP repair over open repair include a reduced risk of infection, less pain, and a faster recovery time [4]. The procedure typically takes 1–2 h and patients can often return to work and normal activities within a week.

TAPP Vs. TEP

Laparoscopic inguinal hernia repair can be performed using two main techniques: Transabdominal Preperitoneal (TAPP) repair and Totally Extraperitoneal (TEP) repair. In TAPP repair, the surgeon gains access to the hernia site by creating an incision in the abdominal wall and entering the peritoneal cavity. The peritoneum is then lifted off the abdominal wall to create a preperitoneal space where the hernia defect is identified and repaired using a mesh. TAPP repair allows for direct visualization of the hernia defect and adjacent structures, enabling thorough assessment and potential concurrent procedures such as repair of a contralateral hernia or a concurrent intraabdominal condition. In TEP repair, the surgeon accesses the hernia site without entering the peritoneal cavity. Instead, the dissection is performed behind the peritoneum, creating an extraperitoneal space. The hernia defect is repaired with a mesh placed in the extraperitoneal space. TEP repair avoids the potential risks associated with entering the peritoneal cavity and has the advantage of not violating the peritoneum, which may be beneficial in patients with previous intra-abdominal surgeries, as it reduces the risk of intra-abdominal adhesions [5].

Both TAPP and TEP techniques have their advantages and considerations, and the choice between them depends on the surgeon's expertise, patient characteristics, and specific clinical circumstances.

Relevant Anatomy

The inguinal region is the area where the abdomen and thigh meet. The inguinal canal is a natural opening in the abdominal wall that allows the spermatic cord in men and the round ligament in women to pass through and enter the groin. The inguinal canal is lined with transversalis fascia and contains the ilioinguinal nerve.

A hernia in the inguinal region occurs when the contents of the abdomen, usually a portion of the small intestine or preperitoneal fat, protrude through a weak area in the abdominal wall into the inguinal canal. This can result in pain, swelling, and a noticeable bulge in the affected area. Hernias can be classified as indirect or direct based on their location relative to the inguinal canal. Indirect hernias are the most common type and occur when the hernia sac passes through the inguinal canal and into the scrotum in men or the labia in women. Direct hernias occur when the hernia sac protrudes through a defect in the abdominal wall directly into the inguinal canal.

In Laparoscopic Totally Extra-peritoneal Repair, the hernia is repaired from outside of the peritoneum, the thin tissue that lines the abdominal cavity and covers the abdominal organs. This technique involves the creation of a space between the peritoneum and the transversalis fascia, called the pre-peritoneal space, where the hernia repair is performed.

The key anatomic landmarks during Laparoscopic TEP repair include the pubic tubercle, the anterior superior iliac spine (ASIS), and the inferior epigastric vessels extending from the external iliac vessels [6]. The pubic tubercle serves as a reference point for the placement of the mesh, while the neurovascular structures must be avoided to minimize the risk of injury. The surgeon uses the laparoscope to visualize the hernia and surrounding structures and to ensure that the mesh is positioned correctly within the pre-peritoneal space. The mesh is then secured in place using sutures or tacks to reinforce the weak area of the abdominal wall and prevent further protrusion of the intestine.

Indications

Laparoscopic Totally Extra-Peritoneal Repair is indicated for the repair of primary and recurrent inguinal hernias in adults [7]. The primary goal of the procedure is to relieve symptoms and prevent the incarceration or strangulation of the hernia, which can result in the loss of blood supply to the herniated intestine.

Patient factors that are good candidates for Laparoscopic TEP repair include bilateral inguinal hernias, recurrent hernia with a previous history of open inguinal hernia repair, and a smaller defect that is fully reducible [8]. The procedure is well-suited for patients who are looking for a minimally invasive alternative to open hernia repair, as it results in less pain, scarring, and a faster recovery time.

It is important to note that not all hernias are suitable for Laparoscopic TEP repair, and a thorough evaluation by a qualified surgeon is necessary to determine the best course of treatment. Factors such as the size and location of the hernia, the patient's overall health, and the surgeon's experience and expertise can all play a role in the decision-making process. Morbidly obese patients, or patients with a history of a prior preperitoneal surgery or midline abdominal surgery, as well as those with a large partially reducible defect, might be better suited with a transabdominal preperitoneal (TAPP) approach. Patients with a history of a previous laparoscopic inguinal repair or prostatectomy, medical conditions that would be a contraindication for general anesthesia with insufflation of the abdominal cavity, and large non-reducible defects would be better suited with an open approach.

Positioning

The patient is positioned supine on the operating table with both arms tucked. Bilateral sequential compression devices are placed on the lower extremities. General anesthesia is administered. A Foley is not routinely placed, with exceptions made for a history of retention, previous inguinal/pelvic surgery, or if there is an anticipated increased length of the procedure. The patient is secured with pressure points padded to minimize the risk of nerve injury or pressure ulcers. The hair of the groin and abdomen is clipped, and the area is prepped with chlorhexidine or isopropyl alcohol. The area is widely draped, leaving the entire abdomen exposed in case of needing to decompress the abdominal cavity and any other variations to the procedure. The surgeon typically stands on the side of the patient contralateral to the hernia.

Access and Trocar Placement

Access to the preperitoneal space is performed via a cut-down technique. A 2-cm infraumbilical incision is made and using electrocautery dissection, the subcutaneous fat and tissue is divided and retracted with S-shaped or Army-Navy retractors. The anterior rectus sheath is exposed and incised off the midline towards the side of the hernia to fit a 12 mm trocar. The rectus muscle is then split with S retractors and retracted laterally to expose the posterior rectus sheath [9].

15 Totally Extraperitoneal Hernia Repair

Technique

A balloon dissector is inserted and carefully advanced in a twisting motion directed inferiorly toward the pubic symphysis while making sure not to violate the intraperitoneal space. A 30-degree laparoscope is inserted, and the balloon is inflated under direct vision in the preperitoneal space. The balloon is then removed and inspected for integrity. The structural balloon trocar is inflated, and CO_2 insufflation of 15 mmHg is started. Two additional 5 mm trocars are inserted in the midline: The second 1 mm above the pubic symphysis and the third midway between the first and second trocars. The inferior epigastric vessels are identified. Dissection is started in the midline, identifying the pubic symphysis, and proceeds laterally to identify the pubic tubercle and Cooper's ligament. The direct space is evaluated and any sac or preperitoneal fat is reduced. The indirect space was then evaluated, and any sac is reduced. There is oftentimes a cord lipoma which is also reduced and separated from the cord structures (Fig. 15.1). The spermatic cord is then skeletonized and separated carefully from any adhered hernia sac, taking care to protect the vas deferens, and pampiniform plexus, as well as avoid the deep vessels (Figs. 15.2, 15.3, 15.4, 15.5, 15.6, 15.7, 15.8, 15.9, and 15.10). If there are bilateral hernias, the dissection is repeated on the contralateral side.

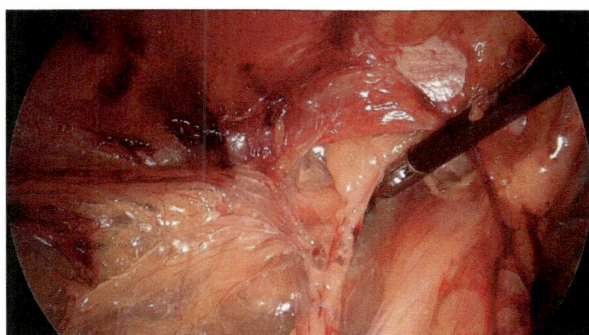

Fig. 15.1 Cord lipoma lateral to the spermatic cord

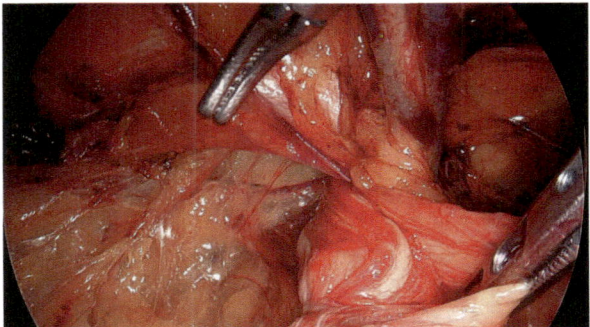

Fig. 15.2 Vas deferens along the spermatic cord visualized

Fig. 15.3 The cord lipoma is grasped and reduced

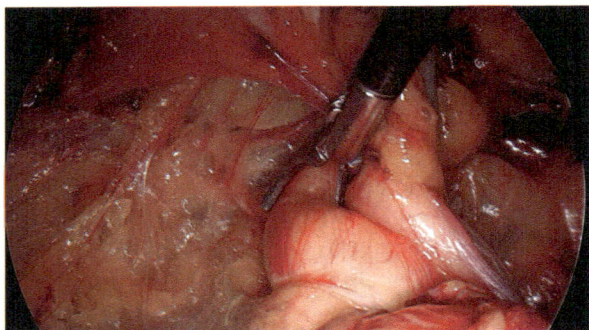

Fig. 15.4 The sac is placed on tension and attachments to the hernia sac are separated

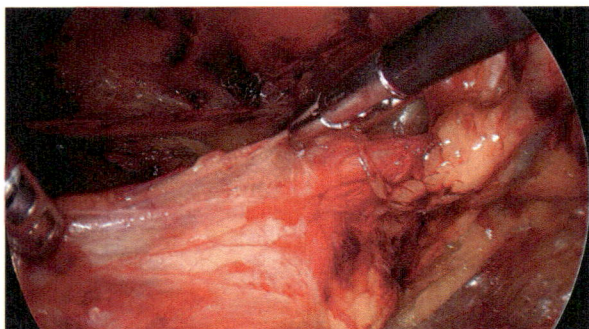

Fig. 15.5 Attachments to the sac are peeled off

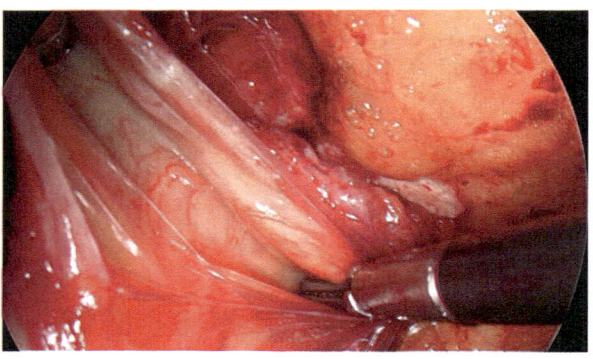

A Dextile 10 × 15 cm mesh is rolled tightly and introduced through the 12 trocar into the preperitoneal space. It is splayed over the myopectineal orifice to lie flush against the tissue and cover the direct, indirect, and femoral spaces. The mesh is secured with a minimal amount of absorbable Vicryl tacks. 1 tack is placed next to

Fig. 15.6 The sac is encircled circumferentially

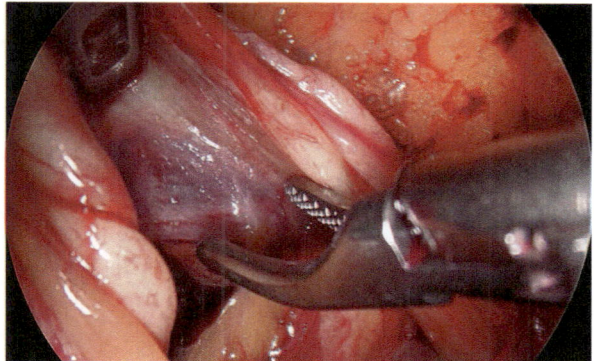

Fig. 15.7 The encircled portion of the sac is placed on tension allowing the distal aspect to be separated from the remaining attachments

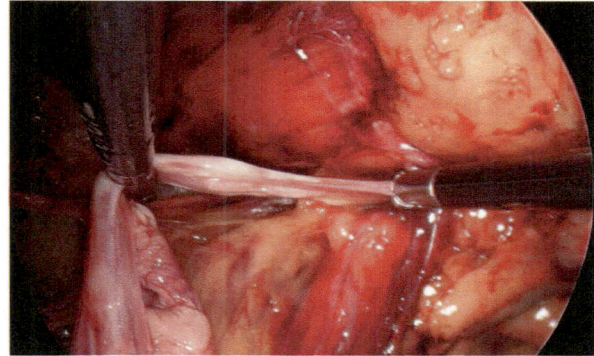

Fig. 15.8 The remaining attachments of the sac to the deep tissue are released

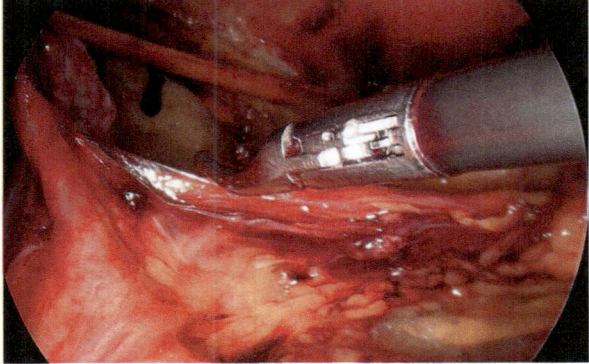

Fig. 15.9 A small hole in the sac is closed with an endoloop

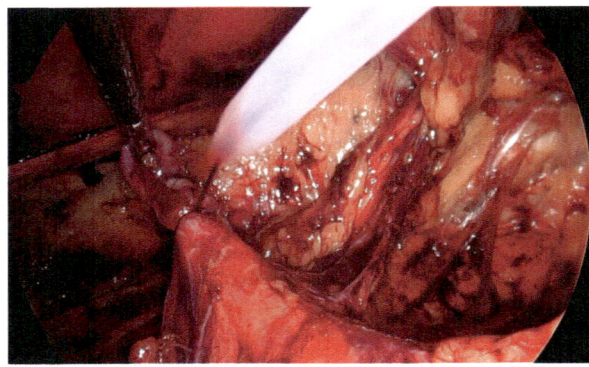

Fig. 15.10 The entire myopectineal orifice is visualized

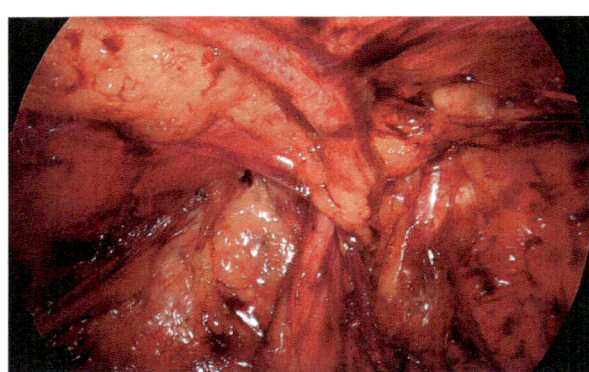

Fig. 15.11 The mesh is tacked at the pubic tubercle

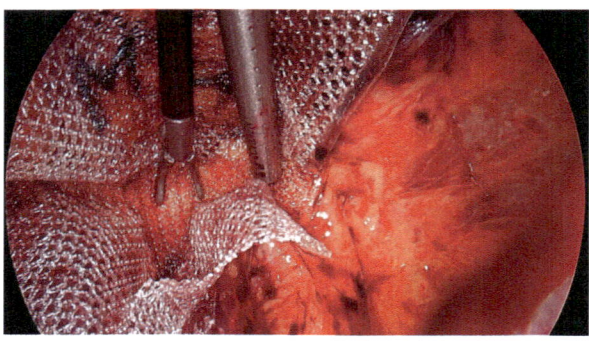

Cooper's ligament (Fig. 15.11). Another tack is placed in the anterior lateral abdominal fascia (Fig. 15.12). An additional tack can be placed superiorly in the midline taking care to avoid epigastric vessels (Fig. 15.13). Two open graspers were used to secure the mesh in place while the abdomen is desufflated under direct visualization (Fig. 15.14).

Fig. 15.12 The mesh is tacked superolaterally (optional)

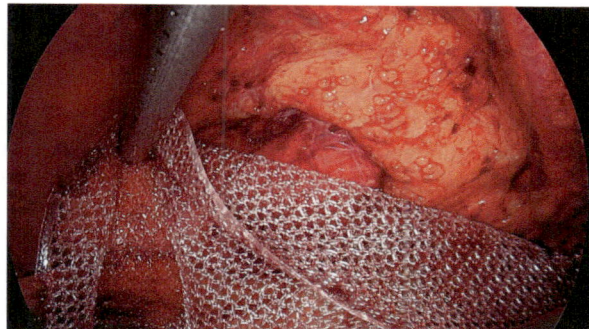

Fig. 15.13 The mesh is tacked superomedially (optional)

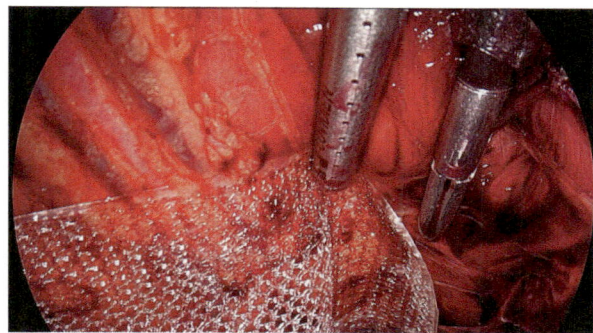

Fig. 15.14 The mesh is held in place with 2 widely opened graspers and the field is desufflated

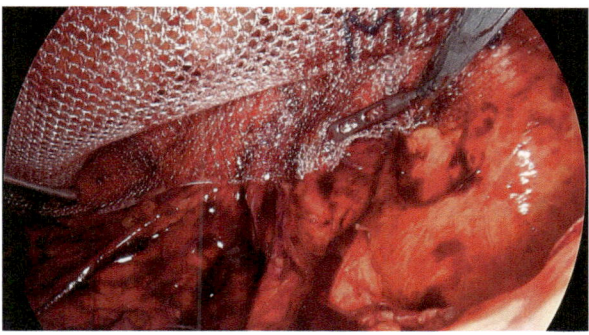

The trocars are then withdrawn. If there was excess intraperitoneal air, the posterior sheath is opened to allow egress of the air and then closed with 0 Vicryl. The anterior sheath is closed with 0 Vicryl and skin incisions are closed with absorbable suture.

Post-operative Care

As with any surgical procedure, Laparoscopic Totally Extra-Peritoneal Repairs carry the risk of potential complications. Some common postoperative complications include seromas, inguinodynia, bleeding, wound complications, and mesh complications such as migration or infection. Patients are counseled about these potential complications in the pre-operative setting. As part of their discharge instructions, they are counseled to contact a physician for symptoms such as fevers/chills, drainage, increased redness or warmth around the incision, and swelling or intractable pain.

Seromas are an anticipated complication that can often be managed with observation. Persistent seromas may require aspiration, which can be performed in the clinic or under ultrasound guidance by interventional radiology. Surgical pain after the procedure is to be anticipated and can be controlled with pain medication. Chronic pain should be approached in a stepwise fashion, with NSAIDs and antispasmodics as ideal first-line treatments. More severe chronic pain may benefit from a referral to a pain specialist for consideration of nerve blocks, and a neurectomy or mesh explantation may need to be considered as a last resort [10]. Local superficial wound infections can be treated by drainage and antibiotics, while deeper mesh complications may require CT scans for further evaluation. In the case of the dreaded mesh infection, a mesh explantation may be required with an expected resulting recurrence of hernia and consideration of a redo repair at a later date.

References

1. Skandalakis L. Hernia History | Atlanta Hernia Surgeon Lee Skandalakis MD FACS. https://herniaspecialists.com/hernia-history/. Accessed 7 Aug 2023.
2. McKernan JB, Laws HL. Laparoscopic repair of inguinal hernias using a totally extraperitoneal prosthetic approach. Surg Endosc. 1993;7(1):26–8.
3. Inguinal Hernia. Inguinal Hernia. http://www.ncbi.nlm.nih.gov/books/NBK513332/. Accessed 7 Aug 2003.
4. Chung RS, Rowland DY. Meta-analyses of randomized controlled trials of laparoscopic vs conventional inguinal hernia repairs. Surg Endosc. 1999;13(7):689–94.
5. Bittner R, Arregui ME, Bisgaard T, et al. Guidelines for laparoscopic (TAPP) and endoscopic (TEP) treatment of inguinal hernia [International Endohernia Society (IEHS)]. Surg Endosc. 2011;25(9):2773–843.
6. Yang XF, Liu JL. Anatomy essentials for laparoscopic inguinal hernia repair. Ann Transl Med. 2016;4(19):372.
7. Hope WW, Pfeifer C. Laparoscopic inguinal hernia repair. [Updated 2023 Feb 8]. In: StatPearls [Internet]. Treasure Island, FL: StatPearls Publishing; 2023. https://www.ncbi.nlm.nih.gov/books/NBK430826/.
8. Cameron JL. Current surgical therapy. 13th ed. Elsevier; 2019.
9. Hoballah JJ, Scott-Conner CEH. Operative dictations in general and vascular surgery. New York, NY: Springer; 2006. https://doi.org/10.1007/978-1-4614-0451-4.
10. Andresen K, Rosenberg J. Management of chronic pain after hernia repair. J Pain Res. 2018;11:675–81.

Index

A
Abdomen, 4, 6, 7, 18–20, 24, 27, 29, 31, 33, 35, 44, 45, 56–58, 72, 80, 89, 95, 111, 130, 132, 134, 141, 150–152, 159, 160, 164
Access
   closed, 99, 151
   open (Hasson), 44, 111, 151
   optical trocar, 44, 132, 151
Anastomotic leak, 35, 58, 93, 108
Anesthesia
   general, 18, 55, 68, 88, 110, 121, 140, 150, 153, 160
   spinal, 88, 121
Anterior resection, 41, 52, 54, 58, 61, 78, 93, 108, 109, 114

B
Bowel preparation, 6, 19, 55, 68, 77, 96, 109, 131, 140

C
Cancer, 24, 33, 73, 77, 88, 94, 95, 97–100, 103, 107–109, 114, 138
Capnoperitoneum, 7, 111, 133, 134, 141, 143
Carcinoma, 3, 18
Circular stapler, 33, 35, 55, 58–60, 80, 81, 113
Clips, 90, 145, 150
Colectomy, 25, 76–78
Colon cancer, 31, 42
Colostomy, 15–21, 52, 65, 67, 68, 72, 73, 138, 139
Conversion, 24, 40, 41, 68, 102, 114, 131, 133

D
da Vinci, 40, 41, 44
Dentate line, 53, 54, 58, 59, 80, 100, 108, 112, 113
Diagnostic laparoscopy, 6, 19, 56, 69, 151
Docking, 40, 44, 99

E
Ergonomics, 40, 91, 151
Extraperitoneal, 21, 138, 145, 158

F
Fibrin glue, 130, 152

G
General, 68

H
Harmonic scalpel, 57, 69, 151
Hemicolectomy, 25, 27–33, 41, 42, 44, 78
Hepatic flexure, 16, 29
Hernia repair, 129, 130, 135, 140, 143, 145, 148, 151, 158–160
Hernia(s), 4, 21, 42, 67, 108, 129, 138, 145
Hybrid, 44, 95
Hypogastric nerve, 76

I
Ileoanal pouch anastomosis (IPAA), 5
Ileocecal valve, 7, 16

Ileocolic artery, 42
Ileostomy, 3–8, 10–12, 18, 21, 52, 78, 79, 81, 114, 138, 139
Indocyanine green (ICG), 29, 58, 59, 72, 113
Inferior mesenteric artery, 31, 69, 78, 111
Inferior mesenteric vein, 32, 57, 69, 111
Inflammatory bowel disease, 11, 67, 76
Informed consent, 6, 18, 55, 98, 109, 131
Inguinal, 130, 131, 145, 146, 148, 149, 151, 158–160

K
Keith needle, 58

L
Laparoscopy, 16, 23, 33, 36, 39, 40, 42, 51, 55, 66, 75, 87, 102, 109, 130, 138, 140, 145, 146, 148, 158
Leak test, 35, 58, 98, 102
Left colic artery, 32, 56, 57, 69
Levator ani, 41, 53, 66, 67, 120
LigaSure, 26, 57, 68, 69, 78
Linear stapler, 33, 35, 68, 80
Lloyd-Davies position, 121
Local excision, 85, 87, 90, 93–95, 97, 100, 101, 103, 109
Loop ileostomy, 3–5, 7, 8, 59, 81
Low anterior, 40, 41, 52, 61

M
Mesh, 21, 41, 43, 72, 119, 123–125, 129–135, 138, 140–143, 145, 150–153, 158, 159, 162, 164–166
Mesocolic excision, 37, 42
Mesorectal fascia, 53, 54, 80
Metastasis, 94, 95, 103
Middle colic artery, 29
Minimally invasive, 23, 51, 66, 75, 90, 91, 94, 107, 158, 160

N
Nervi erigentes, 53, 70, 120, 123

O
Operating room, 19

P
Parastomal, 10, 141, 142
Pneumoperitoneum, 6, 18, 19, 27, 29, 30, 35, 56, 58, 69, 78, 81, 112, 121, 154
Polyps, 54, 87
Port placement, 44–45, 78–80, 111, 151
Proctectomy, 12, 32, 66, 75–80, 98, 109
Proctocolectomy, 109
Prolapse, 3, 4, 10, 11, 21, 42, 125, 140
Purse string, 35, 58, 59, 70, 80, 112, 113

Q
Quality of life, 4, 6, 10, 11, 17, 18, 54, 61, 66, 75, 77, 87, 102, 103, 119

R
Rectal, 5, 18, 23, 39, 51, 65, 76, 77, 80, 85–91, 93–103, 107–109, 112–114, 119, 130
Rectal prolapse, 119
Rectopexy, 41–43, 119, 125
Rectum, 15, 17, 26, 33, 35, 36, 52, 53, 57, 65, 66, 69, 75, 76, 80, 82, 86, 89, 94, 96–98, 102, 111, 113, 119, 120, 122–125
Retroperitoneal, 33, 34, 57, 111, 146, 149
Reverse-Trendelenburg, 57
Revisional surgery, 82, 125
Robot, 37, 39–45, 66, 75, 99, 119, 130
Robot-assisted laparoscopic, 40, 130

S
Sigmoidoscopy, 58, 59, 99, 120
Single incision laparoscopy, 37, 87, 93, 107
Splenic flexure(s), 16, 31–33, 35, 44, 52, 56, 57, 111
Stenosis, 10, 11, 20, 82, 83, 87, 94
Stoma, 3–11, 15–18, 20, 21, 24, 27, 52, 55, 68, 72, 75, 78, 79, 87, 93, 94, 102, 109, 114, 138–141, 143
Stoma prolapse, 21
Stricture, 11, 114
Surgery, 15, 16, 18–21, 52, 66, 75, 88, 93, 107, 129, 140, 145, 158

Index

T
Tacker(s), 143, 150, 152, 153
Totally extraperitoneal, 130, 145, 158, 159, 166
Total mesorectal excision (TME), 41, 44, 52, 65, 100, 107, 114
Transanal endoscopic microsurgery (TEM), 85, 90, 93, 107
Transanal excision, 51, 85–87, 98
Transanal minimally invasive surgery (TAMIS), 87, 90–91, 93, 107
Transanal total mesorectal excision (taTME), 107
Transverse colostomy, 3, 16, 17
Trendelenburg position, 54, 57, 73, 141
Trephine, 4, 8, 9, 29, 138
Trocar(s), 6, 19, 44, 56, 58, 60, 69, 78–81, 96, 109, 111, 112, 131–133, 140–142, 151, 160–162, 165

U
Umbilical ligaments
   lateral, 146
   medial, 146
   median, 146

V
Veress needle, 56, 121, 131

W
Waist' effect, 66

GPSR Compliance

The European Union's (EU) General Product Safety Regulation (GPSR) is a set of rules that requires consumer products to be safe and our obligations to ensure this.

If you have any concerns about our products, you can contact us on ProductSafety@springernature.com

In case Publisher is established outside the EU, the EU authorized representative is:

Springer Nature Customer Service Center GmbH
Europaplatz 3
69115 Heidelberg, Germany

Batch number: 09605312

Printed by Printforce, the Netherlands